Voice Prosthesis in Total Laryngectomized Patients

Springer Nature More Media App

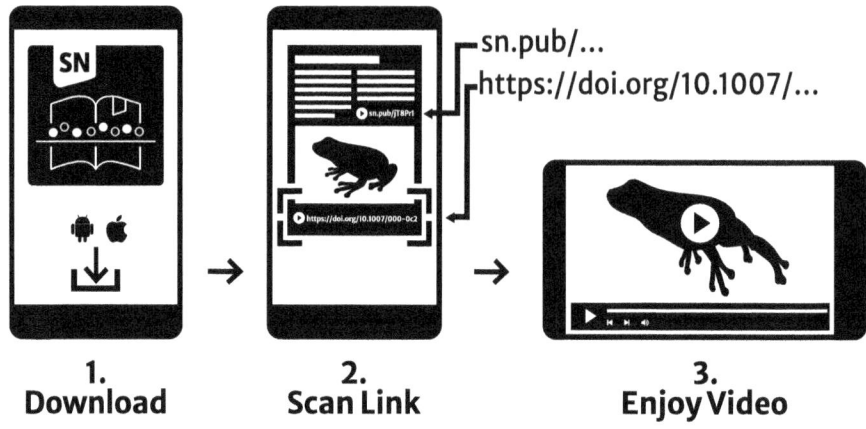

sn.pub/...
https://doi.org/10.1007/...

1.
Download

2.
Scan Link

3.
Enjoy Video

Support: customerservice@springernature.com

Carmelo Saraniti • Barbara Verro
Simona Fiumara

Voice Prosthesis in Total Laryngectomized Patients

From Patient Selection to Complication Management

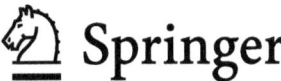

Springer

Carmelo Saraniti
Department of Biomedicine,
Neuroscience and Advanced Diagnostic
University of Palermo
Palermo, Italy

Barbara Verro
Department of Biomedicine,
Neuroscience and Advanced Diagnostic
University of Palermo
Palermo, Italy

Simona Fiumara
Speech therapist
GM Medical
Palermo, Italy

This work contains media enhancements, which are displayed with a "play" icon. Material in the print book can be viewed on a mobile device by downloading the Springer Nature "More Media" app available in the major app stores. The media enhancements in the online version of the work can be accessed directly by authorized users.

ISBN 978-3-031-29656-7   ISBN 978-3-031-29654-3   (eBook)
https://doi.org/10.1007/978-3-031-29654-3

This Springer imprint is published by the registered company Springer Nature Switzerland AG
The registered company address is: Gewerbestrasse 11, 6330 Cham, Switzerland

Paper in this product is recyclable.

Foreword

I was really honored to be asked to write a foreword to this book on *Voice Prosthesis in Total Laryngectomized Patients* written by Professor Carmelo Saraniti, Dr. Barbara Verro both working at the ENT Clinic of the University of Palermo and by Simona Fiumara.

This book faces a very delicate problem as total laryngectomy reduces radically the quality of life and has a great psychological impact on the patients who undergo such a surgical procedure. Since 150 years, when Billroth performed the first total laryngectomy, it became the treatment of choice for advanced laryngeal cancers. In the following years, several more conservative treatments have been proposed according with the localization and the extension of the cancer but the line between the hope to preserve at least partially the quality of life of such patients and the oncological radicality has always been rather uncertain. Moreover, several non-surgical treatments have been proposed in order to preserve the anatomy of the upper respiratory tract but not always these procedures preserved the functions of such a delicate district. Therefore, even today we often have to proceed in most of the T3 and T4 cases to a total laryngectomy, and we must operate in salvage setting also several patients who underwent the protocols for organ preservation.

People who undergo total laryngectomy claim mainly for the presence of the permanent tracheostoma but mainly for the loss of their voice which enables them to communicate.

Therefore, since the 1960s of the last century several surgical procedures have been proposed in order to create a passage (fistula) between trachea and esophagus allowing to the air column produced by the lungs to pass in the esophagus and to be articulated through the remaining part of the vocal tract. Such voice seemed to be of much better quality if compared to the esophageal voice or to electrolarynx which were the only ways at that time to communicate.

Unfortunately, none of them succeeded because of the aspiration. Therefore, in the last two decades of the last century some voice prostheses began to be produced allowing a permanent fistula between the trachea and the esophagus without aspiration.

Such voice prosthesis who underwent during time consistent improvements have gained a great interest and are today considered the gold standard for people who undergo total laryngectomy. Though they may have some complications and they need strict observation in order to maintain their function thus resulting to be very demanding for doctors and speech pathologists that follow such patients.

Prof. Saraniti and his coworkers analyzed in this very interesting and didactic book all the aspects concerning this topic beginning with the selection of patients, the surgical techniques, the timing, the troubleshooting of complications, the office replacement of the prosthesis, and ending with pulmonary rehabilitation, often neglected in laryngectomized patients.

I am sure that this complete overview of the problems concerning the actual rehabilitation will be very useful for those who face the everyday problems of laryngectomized patients helping them to conduct a life as normal as possible despite the very serious handicap caused by the necessary radical surgery.

For this reason, I really thank the Authors and I hope a great success of this publication.

Rome, Italy   Gaetano Paludetti

Contents

1 Introduction... 1
  1.1 Background 1
  1.2 Problems Related to Total Laryngectomy 4
  1.3 Types of Voice Rehabilitation 5
    1.3.1 Esophageal Speech................................. 5
    1.3.2 Electrolarynx 6
    1.3.3 Voice Prosthesis 6
  References... 8

2 Selection: Patient, Surgical Techniques, and Timing............... 11
  2.1 Patient Selection: Who?................................. 11
  2.2 Primary TEP vs. Secondary TEP: Who, When, and Why 13
  2.3 TEP-Related Complications.............................. 15
  2.4 Conclusions 16
  References... 16

3 Surgical Techniques 19
  3.1 Primary Tracheoesophageal Puncture 19
    3.1.1 Section of Trachea/Trachea Dissection 19
    3.1.2 Neurotomy of Monolateral Pharyngeal Plexus and/or
           Monolateral Cricopharyngeal Muscle Myotomy............ 20
    3.1.3 Pharyngeal Suture 22
    3.1.4 Flattening and Stability of Tracheostoma 23
    3.1.5 Techniques for the TEP and Voice Prosthesis Placement 27
  3.2 Secondary TEP... 28
    3.2.1 Complications of the Secondary TEP 31
  References... 31

4 Complications 35
  4.1 Background 35
  4.2 Complications Related to TEP............................. 35
    4.2.1 Enlargement of the TEP............................. 36
    4.2.2 TEP Tract Hypertrophy/Stricture....................... 38
    4.2.3 Granulation Tissue................................. 39
    4.2.4 Peri-prosthetic Bleeding............................ 41

4.2.5   Aspiration or Ingestion of Voice Prosthesis 42
4.2.6   Too Low or Too High TEP 43
4.3   Complications Related to Voice Prosthesis 44
4.3.1   Incontinence of Voice Prosthesis
(Trans-prosthetic Leakage) 44
4.4   Complications Not Related to TEP or Voice Prosthesis 48
4.4.1   Pharyngeal Stricture/Stenosis/Spasm 48
4.4.2   Narrow Tracheostoma 48
4.4.3   Deep Tracheostoma 51
4.5   Troubles in Voice Emission 53
4.5.1   Excessive Length of Voice Prosthesis 53
4.5.2   Short Voice Prosthesis 54
4.5.3   Pharyngeal Hypertonicity 56
4.5.4   Pharyngoesophageal Hypotonia 57
4.5.5   Pressure Sores or Necrosis of the Posterior
Esophageal Wall 58
References 59

5   In-Office Replacement of Voice Prosthesis 63
5.1   Introduction 63
5.2   Pre-operative Evaluation 64
5.3   Voice Prosthesis Replacement Set 65
5.4   Preparation of the Patients 66
5.5   Method of VP Replacement 66
5.5.1   Anterograde Replacement Mode 66
5.5.2   Retrograde Replacement Mode 68
5.6   Final Check 69
References 69

6   Rehabilitation After Total Laryngectomy 71
6.1   Introduction 71
6.2   Respiratory and Pulmonary Rehabilitation 72
6.2.1   Muscle and Pragmatic Relaxation Exercises 77
6.3   Phonatory Rehabilitation 82
6.3.1   Phonatory Rehabilitation Sessions 83
6.3.2   Public Speaking 86
6.4   Rehabilitation of the Sense of Smell 88
6.4.1   The NAIM Manoeuvre 88
References 90

7   Conclusions 93

List of Videos

Video 3.1 Monolateral cricopharyngeal muscle myotomy
Video 3.2 Suture between lower cervical skin flap, sternocleidomastoid muscle, and tracheal ring
Video 3.3 Primary TEP with Provox® voice prosthesis
Video 3.4 Primary TEP with Blom-Singer® voice prosthesis
Video 3.5 Secondary TEP using rigid esophagoscope and Provox® insertion kit
Video 3.6 Secondary TEP using rigid esophagoscope and Blom-Singer® insertion kit (vision from inside)
Video 3.7 Secondary TEP using Yankauer suction tube and Provox® insertion kit
Video 4.1 Tracheal flange colonization with trans-prosthetic leakage
Video 4.2 Intra-esophageal pressure changes synchronous with breathing (tracheal view)
Video 4.3 Intra-esophageal pressure changes synchronous with breathing (esophageal view)

1.1 Background

The first surgeon to successfully perform a total laryngectomy on a human patient was Christian Albert Theodor Billroth who, in 1873, performed this surgery on a 36-year-old man with laryngeal cancer. Only a year later, in 1874, his assistant, Gussenbauer [1] created the first prototype for the restoration of the speech function of laryngectomized patients. Gussenbauer's project involved a device consisting of three cannulas: a tracheal cannula, a pharyngeal cannula, and a voice cannula capable of producing sound through a metal reed. In this way, the occlusion of the cannula with the finger allowed: the passage of air from the trachea to the pharynx, the vibration of the metal reed, and thus, the sound production at the base of the tongue. Moreover, a metal structure at the end of the pharyngeal cannula acted as an epiglottis in order to prevent aspiration. From this primordial idea, various devices and mechanisms have been developed over the decades and numerous surgeries have been carried out with the dual purpose of restoring the speech function and, at the same time, protecting the laryngectomized patient from any tracheal aspirations. Phonation physiology is the basic assumption, from which all the ideas and projects such as Gussebauer's prototype have sprung out over time. Indeed, the production of sound requires three essential elements: the producer of air (lungs), the vibrating structure (larynx), and the articulation system (pharynx and oral cavity). In a healthy subject during phonation, the air from the lungs reaches the larynx where adduction of the vocal cords leads to their vibration and, therefore, the production of a sound which, depending on the movement of the pharyngeal structures, produces the emission of a specific phoneme. Therefore, in the laryngectomized patient, the vibrating structure, that was removed during the surgery, must be restored. Thus, with this assumption and thanks to Gussenbauer's input, various strategies for restoring the vocal tract were proposed.

C. Saraniti et al., *Voice Prosthesis in Total Laryngectomized Patients*, https://doi.org/10.1007/978-3-031-29654-3_1

Furthermore, just as the great discoveries are sometimes the result of chance and unforeseen events, even the speech rehabilitation of the laryngectomized was not without them. In fact, in 1935, Guttmann [2] reported the case of a laryngectomized patient who had created a communication between the trachea and the hypopharynx with an incandescent ice pick. The patient had also come up with a solution to the aspiration problem: occluding the fistula with a goose quill during meals.

This rudimentary idea inspired, about 10 years later, Briani [3] who, through an external valve, put the tracheostoma in direct communication with a fistula made at the esophageal level (1942).

In 1958, Conley [4] improved Briani's design by developing a pharyngocutaneous shunt between esophagus and trachea.

A major breakthrough but simple was the creation of Staffieri [5] who defined it as a *phonatory neoglottis* (1970). This project involved the creation of a tracheopharyngeal fistula through the tubulation of a tract of the hypopharynx mucosa connected to a first small tracheostoma located above a second tracheostoma, intended for breathing.

The pioneer of speech rehabilitation in modern times was Mozolewski [6] who, in 1972, invented the first voice prosthesis consisting of two flanges: a tracheal flange to hold the prosthesis in place and an esophageal flange that ended with a valve in thin polyethylene foil that collapsed during swallowing to avoid aspiration. The prosthesis was placed through retrograde way from the oral cavity. Unfortunately, his invention remained unknown for several years, and Mozolewski did not receive the recognition he well-deserved.

However, his creation helped the speech therapist Blom and the surgeon Singer to develop the *duckbill valves prosthesis* in 1978. The first prototype involved a valve on the esophageal end of the prosthesis. Over the years, Blom and Singer made changes and improvements to this prosthesis: a tracheal flange was added to avoid prosthesis displacement (1981) and the valve was positioned inside the prosthesis tube itself for its better functioning (1883). In 1998, the changes to the tracheal and esophageal flange made the Blom and Singer prosthesis indwelling and positionable through the anterograde way [7] (Fig. 1.1).

In recent decades, the voice prosthesis has undergone further changes in order to improve its features as well as the patient's quality of life, reducing the pressures necessary for phonation, minimizing the risk of microbial colonization of the prosthesis itself, up to the introduction of an automatic valve that allows to speak without using the hand to occlude the tracheal stoma [8].

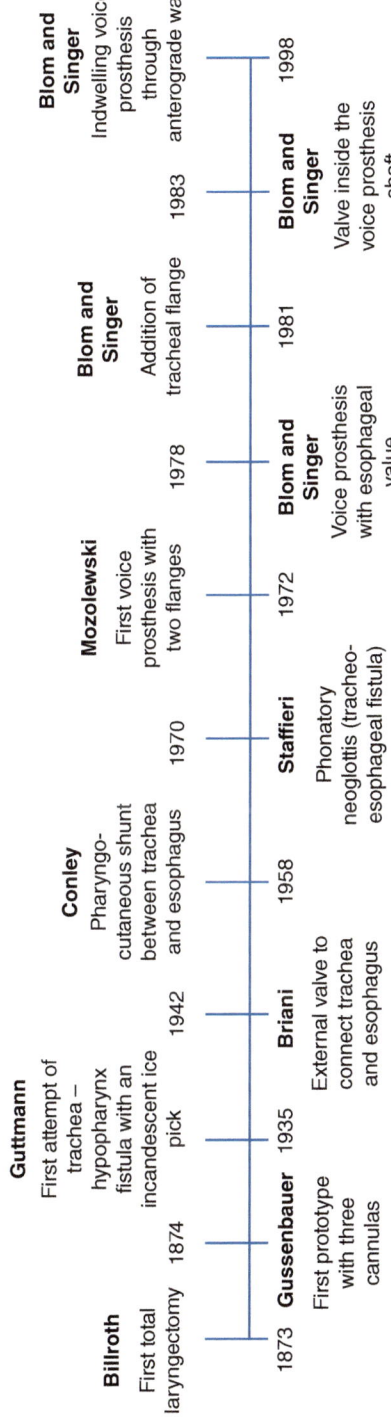

Fig. 1.1 History of voice prosthesis

1.2   Problems Related to Total Laryngectomy

Total laryngectomy represents a real impairment for the patient with a serious impact on his quality of life. In fact, upon awakening from the surgery, the laryngectomized patient experiences three traumas: loss of verbal communication, the presence of a tracheostoma essential for breathing, and lastly, loss of smell.

Loss of speech means communication difficulties with all the resulting consequences: the patient feels alone and misunderstood and ends up isolating himself, creating a vicious circle of depression and loneliness [9]. In fact, as reported by Lorenz et al. the voice helps to define the individual's identity [8]. This explains why, just 1 year after the first total laryngectomy, surgeons immediately thought about how to return the voice to the patient. Indeed, the success of the treatment of laryngeal carcinoma cannot and should not be assessed solely on the basis of the oncological result. Therefore, already in the pre-operative, the existence of different speech rehabilitation strategies is explained to the patient: esophageal voice, electrolarynx, and voice prosthesis. Each one has indications, advantages and disadvantages but, regardless of which type of voice will be used, the patient undergoes the surgery with confidence and hope of speaking again.

In the post-operative, the patient experiences the second trauma: the tracheostoma, which is the circular slot on the neck that allows him to breathe and that will accompany him throughout his life. The tracheostoma has a dual impact: it alters the physiology of breathing and, even more seriously, it worsens the quality of life of the subject who perceives the stoma as a stigma that he cannot hide or remove. Therefore, the patient must begin a real path of acceptance of tracheostoma: looking in the mirror, becoming familiar with his stoma, learning to independently manage the toilet of the cannula, the prosthesis, and the peristomal skin itself. It is more difficult to accept the glances of others, passers-by or acquaintances who stare at the stoma with curiosity, compassion, or repulsion. Because of this, laryngectomized patients sometimes implement strategies to hide the stoma, such as using a scarf around the neck. In addition to the psychological impact, it is also necessary to consider the respiratory changes that derive from creating a direct communication between the external environment and the lower airways (LA) without the filter and barrier function generally performed by the upper airways (nose, mouth, larynx) (UA). In fact, the hair cells and goblet cells that make up the respiratory epithelium perform an important protective function of the LA, thanks to the action of so-called *muco-ciliary clearance*, as well as humidification of the air that reaches the bronchi. Therefore, on the one hand, the mucus produced by the goblet cells traps any particles and microorganisms and, on the other hand, the cilia of the respiratory mucosa, with their coordinated movement, facilitate their elimination in the digestive tract or directly in the external environment. Moreover, the nose and, in general, the UA also perform a humidification function of the inspired air which, once it reaches the trachea, will have a temperature of about 30–32 °C and a relative humidity of up to 99%. However, in the laryngectomized patient, the humidification function is substituted by the respiratory tracheobronchial epithelium which not only fails to obtain optimal temperature and humidity of the inspired air but, above all, in this attempt, compromises the quality of the muco-ciliary clearance with dehydration of the epithelium and increased mucus production. This results in reduced mucus fluidity with the formation of mucus plugs that promote microbial growth [10]. The body tries to defend itself through the cough reflex which, however, is ineffective and causes irritation of the tracheobronchial mucosa, establishing a vicious circle that compromises lung function and, therefore, the patient's quality of life. For this reason, the use of the Heat and Moisture Exchanger (HME) filter is important and fundamental for the laryngectomized because it takes over the function of humidification and filter of the inspired air [11, 12]. Thus, the patient must be educated and made aware of the constant use of the filter, once again focusing attention on the ultimate goal of speech and pulmonary rehabilitation of the laryngectomized, thus ensuring a good quality of life.

Finally, total laryngectomy also involves a progressive reduction or complete loss of the sense of smell. Indeed, the lack of air flow through the nose over time causes atrophy of the nasal mucosa and degeneration of the neuroepithelium of the olfactory bulb with consequent hyposmia or anosmia [13]. Sometimes, albeit less frequently, an impairment of the sense of taste is also associated. In a 2014 study, Mumovic et al. found hyposmia and anosmia in 51.4% and 30.5% of the recruited laryngectomized patients respectively; hypogeusia was instead reported by 26.7% of the patients [14]. These disorders are inevitably responsible for a deterioration in the quality of life. To date, the aspect of anosmia is often considered secondary in the rehabilitation of the laryngectomized patient; instead, the sense of smell plays a role of primary importance in many aspects of everyday life. For this reason, in the last 20 years, various strategies and techniques for olfactory rehabilitation have been proposed. To date, the best known and most effective technique is the Polite Yawning Technique or Nasal Airflow-Inducing Maneuver which has been shown to be able to guarantee the recovery of smell in about 50% of laryngectomized patients [15].

1.3   Types of Voice Rehabilitation

1.3.1   Esophageal Speech

Described for the first time by Strubing and Landois in 1889 [16], the esophageal speech represents the most "natural" phonatory technique. In fact, it is produced through the ingestion of air in the esophagus which, at a later time, is released in a measured and controlled way, causing the vibration of the pharyngo-esophageal tract, defined as "pseudoglottis" by Seemann [17]. Then, depending on the movement of the joint system (pharynx and oral cavity), the mucosa's vibration is transformed into a specific phoneme. Therefore, it represents an advantageous speech technique for two main reasons: it does not require further surgical interventions and has no cost as residual anatomical structures and para-physiological mechanisms are used (belching) [8].

The only contraindications are hypertonicity of the cricopharyngeal muscle and the presence of pharyngeal and/or esophageal stenosis. In this case, it will be necessary to perform surgery or to inject botulinum toxin to eliminate this obstacle to phonation [9]. Furthermore, it should be emphasized that the esophageal speech, despite exploiting a "natural reflex," has two main limitations: firstly, the technique itself requires a frequent supply of air in the esophagus, making fluent speech difficult; secondly, it has a long and difficult learning curve and only a small percentage of laryngectomized learn to use this voice. To confirm this, in 2004, Van As et al. reported that one-third of laryngectomized patients could use their esophageal voice and that only 10% of them spoke clearly [18].

1.3.2   Electrolarynx

Another speech technique, introduced at the end of the 1920s, is the so-called electrolarynx which consists of the vibration—at a constant fundamental frequency—of the mucous membrane of pharynx thanks to an external device: the laryngophone. In particular, there are three types of laryngophones: external transcervical, external transoral, and intraoral devices. To date, the external transcervical laryngophone is the most used and it can be positioned on the neck, at the neopharynx, or under the mandible at the oral floor, thus determining the vibration of the pharyngeal mucosa or of the oral cavity, respectively [8].

Therefore, the production of this voice does not require any specific surgical intervention and, unlike the esophageal speech, it is easy to understand and use.

In any case, these advantages are contrasted by two main problems: the metallic voice, without variations in the voice's tone, and the need to always keep the laryngophone in hand. In fact, several studies have shown that the metallic voice of the electrolarynx is associated with a greater perception of the vocal handicap by the patient, when compared to the tracheoesophageal puncture (TEP), both as regard to the voice's tone and the speech intelligibility, especially for deaf consonants (t, p, k). Finally, a basic requirement for the operation of the device is the integrity of the articulation system which can be compromised in the case of an enlarged total laryngectomy [9, 19]. Therefore, the electrolarynx is indicated as a "rescue" option in the case of laryngectomized patients who cannot use the voice prosthesis and who are unable to speak with the esophageal speech.

1.3.3   Voice Prosthesis

The voice prosthesis represents the gold standard for the voice rehabilitation of the laryngectomized as it restores the physiology of phonation. Indeed, the air from the lungs goes up into the trachea and from here, through a communication created surgically between the posterior tracheal wall and the anterior esophageal wall, reaches the pharynx and oral cavity, allowing the emission of phonemes. The voice prosthesis is placed in this fistula, so-called TEP, in order to direct the air into the esophagus only at the time of speech and, at the same time, protect the airways from possible ab-ingestis thanks to a one-way valve placed inside it [9].

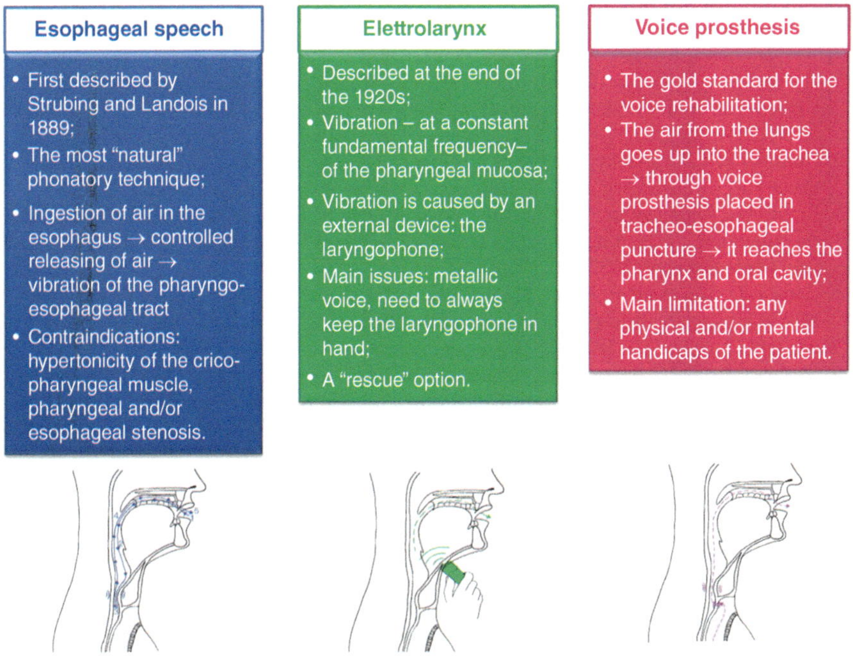

Esophageal speech	Elettrolarynx	Voice prosthesis
• First described by Strubing and Landois in 1889; • The most "natural" phonatory technique; • Ingestion of air in the esophagus → controlled releasing of air → vibration of the pharyngo-esophageal tract • Contraindications: hypertonicity of the crico-pharyngeal muscle, pharyngeal and/or esophageal stenosis.	• Described at the end of the 1920s; • Vibration – at a constant fundamental frequency– of the pharyngeal mucosa; • Vibration is caused by an external device: the laryngophone; • Main issues: metallic voice, need to always keep the laryngophone in hand; • A "rescue" option.	• The gold standard for the voice rehabilitation; • The air from the lungs goes up into the trachea → through voice prosthesis placed in tracheo-esophageal puncture → it reaches the pharynx and oral cavity; • Main limitation: any physical and/or mental handicaps of the patient.

Fig. 1.2 Types of voice rehabilitation

By comparing the three voice rehabilitation techniques, several studies have demonstrated and established the superiority of the voice prosthesis in terms of voice quality and, consequently, life's quality. Moreover, it is possible to perform the surgery to create the tracheoesophageal fistula and place a voice prosthesis both at the same time of the total laryngectomy (primary technique) or later (secondary technique), based on the choice of the surgeon and the patient [20]. It is important to emphasize that adjuvant radiotherapy and/or the use of microsurgical free flap for the reconstruction of the pharynx after total laryngectomy are not contraindications to the positioning of the voice prosthesis [21, 22].

The main limitation to TEP is represented by any physical and/or mental handicaps of the patient (stroke, amputations of the upper limbs, severe respiratory insufficiency, etc.) which prevent the closure of the stoma or the respiration-phonation coordination. In addition, unlike the esophageal speech and electrolarynx, the voice prosthesis requires daily management and maintenance as well as its outpatient replacement about 3–4 times a year.

Overall, therefore, the voice prosthesis represents the first-choice technique for voice rehabilitation since it allows a satisfactory recovery of the voice, in terms of quality and intelligibility, with a rapid learning of its functioning which is almost "natural" (Fig. 1.2).

Declaration by Authors Figures are original and free from copyright issues.

References

1. Gussenbauer C. Ueber die erste durch Th. Billroth am Menschen ausgeführte Kehlkopf—
   Exstirpation und die Anwendung eines künstlichen Kehlkopfes. Arch Klin Chir Berlin.
   1874;17:343–56.
2. Guttman MR. Tracheohypopharyngeal fistulation. A new procedure for speech production in
   the laryngectomized patient. Trans Am Laryngol Rhinol Otol Soc. 1935;41:219–26.
3. Briani AA. Riabilitazione fonetica di laringectomizzati a mezzo della corrente aerea espirato-
   ria polmonare [Speech rehabilitation in laryngectomized by means of expired air]. Arch Ital
   Otol Rinol Laringol. 1952;63(5):469–75.
4. Conley JJ, Deamesti F, Pierce MK. A new surgical technique for the vocal rehabilitation
   of the laryngectomized patient. Ann Otol Rhinol Laryngol. 1958;67(3):655–64. https://doi.
   org/10.1177/000348945806700306.
5. Staffieri M. Funktionelle totale Laryngektomie. Total functional laryngectomy. Surgical technic, indications and results of a personal technic for glottis-plasty with reconstruction of the
   voice. Monatsschr Ohrenheilkd Laryngorhinol. 1973;107(2):77–89.
6. Mozolewski E, Zietek E, Jach K. Surgical rehabilitation of voice and speech after laryngectomy. Pol Med Sci Hist Bull. 1973;15(4):373–7.
7. Blom ED. Tracheoesophageal voice restoration: origin—evolution—state-of-the-art. Folia
   Phoniatr Logop. 2000;52(1–3):14–23. https://doi.org/10.1159/000021508.
8. Lorenz KJ. Rehabilitation after total laryngectomy—a tribute to the pioneers of voice restoration in the last two centuries. Front Med (Lausanne). 2017;4:81. https://doi.org/10.3389/
   fmed.2017.00081.
9. Tang CG, Sinclair CF. Voice restoration after total laryngectomy. Otolaryngol Clin N Am.
   2015;48(4):687–702. https://doi.org/10.1016/j.otc.2015.04.013.
10. Rosso M, Prgomet D, Marjanović K, Pušeljić S, Kraljik N. Pathohistological changes of tracheal
    epithelium in laryngectomized patients. Eur Arch Otorrinolaringol. 2015;272(11):3539–44.
    https://doi.org/10.1007/s00405-014-3396-5.
11. Wong CY, Shakir AA, Farboud A, Whittet HB. Active versus passive humidification for self-
    ventilating tracheostomy and laryngectomy patients: a systematic review of the literature. Clin
    Otolaryngol. 2016;41(6):646–51. https://doi.org/10.1111/coa.12577.
12. Quail G, Fagan JJ, Raynham O, Krynauw H, John LR, Carrara H. Effect of cloth stoma covers
    on tracheal climate of laryngectomy patients. Head Neck. 2016;38(Suppl 1):E480–7. https://
    doi.org/10.1002/hed.24022.
13. Veyseller B, Ozucer B, Aksoy F, Yildirim YS, Gurbuz D, Balikci HH, et al. Reduced olfac-
    tory bulb volume and diminished olfactory function in total laryngectomy patients: a pro-
    spective longitudinal study. Am J Rhinol Allergy. 2012;26(3):191–3. https://doi.org/10.2500/
    ajra.2012.26.3768.
14. Mumovic G, Hocevar-Boltezar I. Olfaction and gustation abilities after a total laryngectomy.
    Radiol Oncol. 2014;48(3):301–6. https://doi.org/10.2478/raon-2013-0070.
15. Hilgers FJ, van Dam FS, Keyzers S, Koster MN, van As CJ, Muller MJ. Rehabilitation of olfac-
    tion after laryngectomy by means of a nasal airflow-inducing maneuver: the "polite yawning"
    technique. Arch Otolaryngol Head Neck Surg. 2000;126(6):726–32. https://doi.org/10.1001/
    archotol.126.6.726.
16. Struebing PL, Landois L. Erzeugung einer (natürlichen) Pseudo-Stimme bei einem Manne mit
    totaler Extirpation des Kehlkopfes. Arch Klin Chir. 1889;38:143.
17. Seemann M. Phoniatrische Bemerkungen zur Laryngektomie. Arch Klin Chir.
    1926;140:285–98.
18. Van As CJ, Op De Coul BM, Eysholdt U, Hilgers FJ. Value of digital high-speed endoscopy
    in addition to videofluoroscopic imaging of the neoglottis in tracheoesophageal speech. Acta
    Otolaryngol. 2004;124(1):82–9. https://doi.org/10.1080/00016480310015290.

19. Kaye R, Tang CG, Sinclair CF. The electrolarynx: voice restoration after total laryngectomy. Med Devices (Auckl). 2017;10:133–40. Published 2017 Jun 21. https://doi.org/10.2147/MDER.S133225.
20. Elmiyeh B, Dwivedi RC, Jallali N, Chisholm EJ, Kazi R, Clarke PM, et al. Surgical voice restoration after total laryngectomy: an overview. Indian J Cancer. 2010;47(3):239–47. https://doi.org/10.4103/0019-509X.64707.
21. Massaro N, Verro B, Greco G, Chianetta E, D'Ecclesia A, Saraniti C. Quality of life with voice prosthesis after total laryngectomy. Iran J Otorhinolaryngol. 2021;33(118):301–9. https://doi.org/10.22038/ijorl.2021.53724.2832.
22. Sinclair CF, Rosenthal EL, McColloch NL, Magnuson JS, Desmond RA, Peters GE, et al. Primary versus delayed tracheoesophageal puncture for laryngopharyngectomy with free flap reconstruction. Laryngoscope. 2011;121(7):1436–40. https://doi.org/10.1002/lary.21836.

Selection: Patient, Surgical Techniques, and Timing

Key Points

- The indication to voice prosthesis rehabilitation depends on several patient-related factors.
- Patient selection for TEP is an important moment that requires a multidisciplinary team.
- The choice of primary or secondary TEP should be also assessed based on many factors.
- Overall, primary TEP should be preferred.
- Secondary TEP is recommended in case of reconstruction with free flap or previous radiotherapy.
- There are general rules but they must be tailored to the individual patient.

2.1   Patient Selection: Who?

To date, the voice prosthesis (VP) is considered the gold standard for speech rehabilitation in patients undergoing total laryngectomy. However, its positioning and use have indications and contraindications, so it is essential to carefully select the patient. Before the creation of a tracheoesophageal puncture (TEP) for indwelling prosthesis, the patient and his family surroundings should be assessed. For this purpose, several medical figures are involved, first the *otolaryngologist* [1]. The patient and his family should come back into contact with the otolaryngologist who diagnosed the tumor, so he may provide all the necessary information about the total laryngectomy surgery and the possibility to place the VP, simultaneously or later. Thus, the ENT specialist is the first filter: he knows the patient, his history, his comorbidities and, consequently, he is the first to express an opinion on his candidacy for the speech prosthesis.

© The Author(s), under exclusive license to Springer Nature Switzerland AG 2024
C. Saraniti et al., *Voice Prosthesis in Total Laryngectomized Patients*, https://doi.org/10.1007/978-3-031-29654-3_2

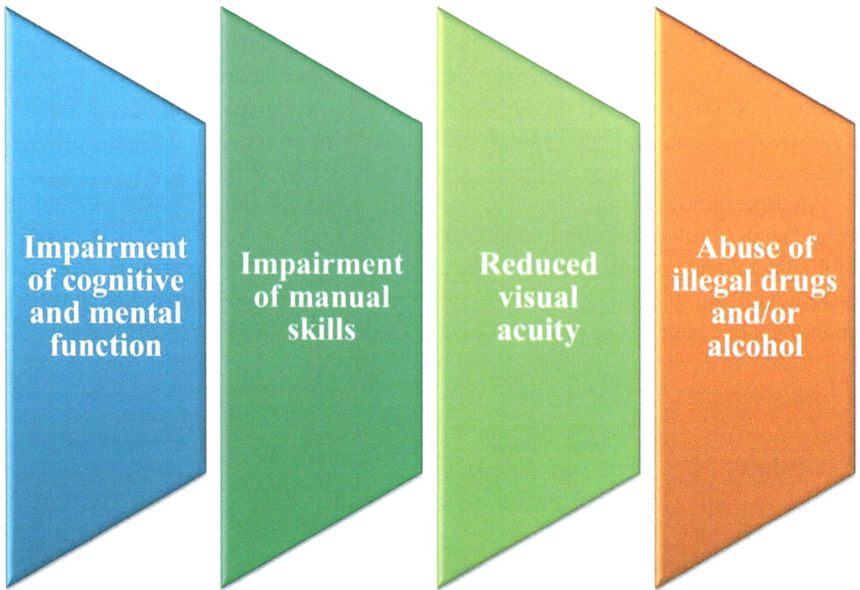

Fig. 2.1 TEP contraindication

Indeed, the first and main contraindication to TEP is impairment of cognitive and mental function as well as manual skills that would not allow the use and the correct and necessary management of the VP of the patient [2, 3] (Fig. 2.1).

The type of demolitive surgery (laryngectomy or pharyngolaryngectomy) to be performed and, therefore, the possible need for reconstruction with pedunculated or free flap [4] do not represent absolute contraindication to the creation of a TEP [5, 6]. Likewise, chemotherapy and/or radiotherapy (RT) do not contraindicate the placement of the VP [7], they may possibly affect the timing of the procedure. Studies have shown that RT does not incur an increased risk of TEP-related complications [1], at most it can shorten the life of the VP [8]. Thus, summing up, the factors that correlate with the success of the TEP are the following: (1) use of the voice prosthesis as a means of communication by the patient (no use, occasional, or common use of the VP); (2) quality of the voice in terms of easy phonation and speech intelligibility; (3) care and management of VP and TEP (daily cleaning of the prosthesis, ability to recognize any TEP-related problems, easy to find the material for the management of the TEP) [9].

Once the suitability of the prosthetic rehabilitation for the patient is established, the surgeon evaluates the opportunity of inserting the prosthesis during the total laryngectomy surgery (primary TEP) or later (secondary TEP).

In the multidisciplinary study of the laryngectomized patient candidate for positioning of the VP, the *pneumonologist* who examines the lung capacity of the patient is also involved in order to determine whether the patient would be able to overcome the resistances and pressures needed for phonation with VP. Indeed, the chronic

Fig. 2.2 TEP candidacy: decision-making

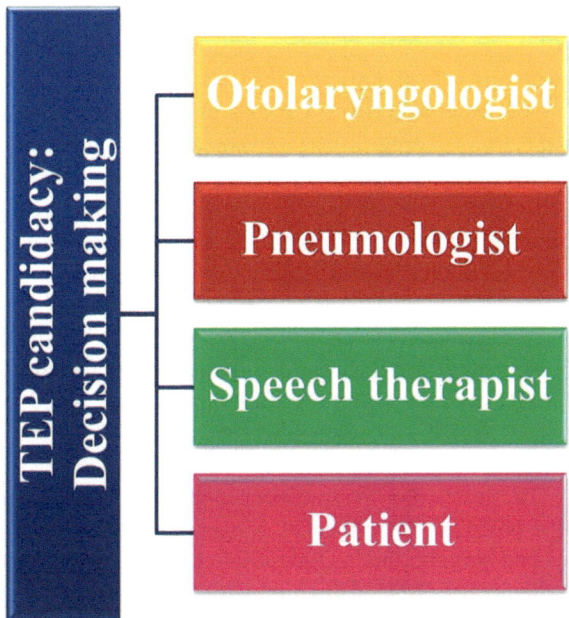

obstructive pulmonary disease (COPD), responsible for severe impairment of respiratory function and increased risk of lung infections, is a common finding in the patient with laryngeal cancer since both diseases recognize smoking as the main risk factor [10]. Thus, in this context, the role of the pulmonologist is important since he studies the patient's respiratory function through the spirometry and adds an additional element for his candidacy or less to TEP.

Another fundamental medical figure is the *speech therapist* that assesses the integrity of the anatomical structures involved in phonation: the emission of air from the lungs, air transmission, and vibration of the pharyngoesophageal tract, articulation of sound through tongue, teeth, and lips [11]. Moreover, the speech therapist researches with more depth the family surroundings and environment and his level of motivation, although the latter is not a decisive requirement for the success of the VP rehabilitation [12] (Fig. 2.2).

2.2 Primary TEP vs. Secondary TEP: Who, When, and Why

As mentioned above, TEP creation could be performed simultaneously with the total laryngectomy surgery (primary TEP) or later (secondary TEP). The choice of timing is determined by several factors dependent on the surgeon, the patient with his comorbidities, and on the cancer in terms of type of surgery performed (possible reconstruction with free flap), any adjuvant therapy, and TNM staging [13].

Several studies have shown that both primary and secondary techniques are effective and safe, with satisfactory results in terms of speech rehabilitation [1, 6,

14]. However, each technique has advantages and disadvantages that make it more or less suitable for some patients rather than for others, although to date this topic is still the matter of debate.

The creation of the tracheoesophageal fistula with placement of VP during the total laryngectomy surgery (*primary TEP*) is advantageous since it allows an early speech rehabilitation and prevents the patient from undergoing a second surgery under general anesthesia. This explains the increased success rate of speech rehabilitation and patient satisfaction with the primary technique as it encourages the motivation and determination of the patient who in fact can starts talking already 2 weeks after total laryngectomy [15]. Moreover, comparison between laryngectomy patients and laryngectomy patients with VP showed no difference in terms of complication rate and length of hospitalization [16]. The only contraindications to the primary TEP are represented by possible damage to the tracheoesophageal wall, that could cause mediastinitis, and by the experience of the surgeon. Therefore, where conditions permit, primary TEP is preferred.

The creation of the tracheoesophageal fistula with *secondary technique* was the first procedure described by Singer and Blom in 1980 [17]. Even if it requires a second surgery, this technique often is indicated when the patient has undergone radiotherapy or reconstruction with free flap.

Indeed, RT is responsible for a weakening of the treated tissues as well as slower healing of the surgical site: these factors correlate to a higher risk of complications, so the creation of the TEP is often postponed at least 4 months after the last radiation therapy session [18]. However, despite in clinical practice, the placement of the VP is usually performed for prophylactic and protective purposes [1, 14], several studies have reported that, in case of salvage total laryngectomy or adjuvant radiotherapy, the success rate of TEP and the risk of complications do not show a statistically significant difference between the primary and secondary technique [6, 16, 19].

As mentioned above, secondary TEP is usually indicated also in situations of reconstruction of the pharynx with microsurgical free flaps [20]. Indeed, in case of pharyngolaryngectomy, in the reconstructive step, free flaps are used, more often the radial forearm fascio-cutaneous flap (RFFF) or the anterolateral thigh flap (ALT). Many studies have been carried out to assess the best choice for these patients between primary and secondary TEP technique, but none showed a real advantage [6], or more precisely, a lower risk of complications between the two surgical procedures [1, 19]. In 2011, Sinclair et al. conducted a study on patients undergoing total laryngectomy and reconstruction with free flap finding primary TEP success in terms of voice quality and voice rehabilitation in two-thirds of the examined patients. Their study also reported a difference in the timing of recovery of phonation with a median time of 56 days in case of primary technique and 200 days in case of secondary technique [20].

A 2008 study analyzed the variable "age" showing that, in patients older than 61 years, secondary TEP correlates with a higher success rate of speech rehabilitation [21] according to the Harrison-Robillard Shultz Tracheoesophageal Puncture Rating Scale (HRS) [9].

Table 2.1 Primary vs secondary TEP

	Primary TEP	Secondary TEP
Pro	• Early speech rehabilitation • Single surgery • Increased success rate of speech rehabilitation • Better patient satisfaction	• Better after pharyngeal reconstruction with free flaps • Better after radiation therapy
Cons	• Possible delayed healing	• Second surgery under general anesthesia • Late recovery of phonation • Increased risk of intra and post-operative complications

Anyway, if the parameter "success of speech rehabilitation" is considered, without distinction of age, free flaps, or any other variables, the current literature agrees in claiming less satisfactory results with the secondary technique, although there is no statistically significant difference between the two procedures. This result could be explained by the late recovery of phonation that first has a negative psychological impact on the patient, but it also relates to a difficulty in changing the mode of phonation in a patient accustomed to speaking with esophageal voice, after ingestion of air. Therefore, in contrast to primary TEP, in this case the patient often needs speech therapist support to be trained on the different phonatory technique (Table 2.1).

2.3   TEP-Related Complications

The creation of a tracheoesophageal fistula with placement of voice prostheses correlates to risk of complications ranging from 15 to 70% [18]. These can be divided into major and minor, whether or not they require surgical resolution, and into direct and indirect if they are directly or indirectly related to the TEP or the VP. Direct complications include the dilation of the TEP with aspiration of the prosthesis and/or peri-prosthetic leakage resulting in aspiration pneumonia, the peri-prosthetic granulation tissue, and partial or complete closure of the TEP. Indirect complications are pharyngo-cutaneous fistula, pharyngeal hypertonia, and tracheostomy stenosis [1]. According to current literature, the risk of developing such complications is overlapping between the primary and secondary TEP technique [1, 14, 19]. In this regard, Barauna Neto et al. have reviewed the literature comparing the two techniques in terms of the incidence of the following complications: infection, tracheostomy stenosis, pharyngo-cutaneous fistula, and peri-prosthetic leakage [15]. Their study showed that the primary technique runs a greater risk of developing these complications but their different incidence between the two techniques is not statistically significant. Pharyngocutaneous fistula seems to occur statistically more often in the case of primary TEP, with an additional increased incidence in the case of salvage total laryngectomy, namely in the case of tissues previously treated with radiotherapy [14, 22, 23].

2.4   Conclusions

In view of the above, proper and careful patient selection for TEP, primary or secondary, is important and fundamental in order to ensure the patient the best voice rehabilitation with a satisfactory quality of life and the lowest possible risk of TEP-related complications. Therefore, whenever possible, a primary TEP should be performed; however, in case of reconstruction with free flap or previous radiotherapy, a secondary TEP is recommended. In fact, as the Latins said, *primum non nocere, secundum cavere, and tertium sanare.*

Declaration by Authors   Figures are original and free from copyright issues.

References

1. Gitomer SA, Hutcheson KA, Christianson BL, Samuelson MB, Barringer DA, Roberts DB, Hessel AC, Weber RS, Lewin JS, Zafereo ME. Influence of timing, radiation, and reconstruction on complications and speech outcomes with tracheoesophageal puncture. Head Neck. 2016;38(12):1765–71. https://doi.org/10.1002/hed.24529. Epub 2016 Jul 9. PMID: 27394060; PMCID: PMC5118069.
2. Wachal B, Johnson M, Burchell A, Sayles H, Rieke K, Lindau R, Lydiatt W, Panwar A. Association of modified Frailty Index Score with perioperative risk for patients undergoing total laryngectomy. JAMA Otolaryngol Head Neck Surg. 2017;143(8):818–23. https://doi.org/10.1001/jamaoto.2017.0412. PMID: 28594992; PMCID: PMC5710554.
3. Kwon JH, Hui D, Chisholm G, Bruera E. Predictors of long-term opioid treatment among patients who receive chemoradiation for head and neck cancer. Oncologist. 2013;18(6):768–74. https://doi.org/10.1634/theoncologist.2013-0001. Epub 2013 May 30. PMID: 23723332; PMCID: PMC4063405.
4. Nguyen S, Thuot F. Functional outcomes of fasciocutaneous free flap and pectoralis major flap for salvage total laryngectomy. Head Neck. 2017;39(9):1797–805. https://doi.org/10.1002/hed.24837. Epub 2017 Jun 5.
5. Revenaugh PC, Knott PD, Alam DS, Kmiecik J, Fritz MA. Voice outcomes following reconstruction of laryngopharyngectomy defects using the radial forearm free flap and the anterolateral thigh free flap. Laryngoscope. 2014;124(2):397–400. https://doi.org/10.1002/lary.23785. Epub 2013 Oct 15.
6. Massaro N, Verro B, Greco G, Chianetta E, D'Ecclesia A, Saraniti C. Quality of life with voice prosthesis after total laryngectomy. Iran J Otorhinolaryngol. 2021;33(118):301–9. https://doi.org/10.22038/ijorl.2021.53724.2832. PMID: 34692577; PMCID: PMC8507945.
7. Boscolo-Rizzo P, Marchiori C, Gava A, Da Mosto MC. The impact of radiotherapy and GERD on in situ lifetime of indwelling voice prostheses. Eur Arch Otorrinolaringol. 2008;265(7):791–6. https://doi.org/10.1007/s00405-007-0536-1. Epub 2007 Nov 16.
8. Elving GJ, Van Weissenbruch R, Busscher HJ, Van Der Mei HC, Albers FW. The influence of radiotherapy on the lifetime of silicone rubber voice prostheses in laryngectomized patients. Laryngoscope. 2002;112(9):1680–3. https://doi.org/10.1097/00005537-200209000-00028.
9. Shultz JR, Harrison J. Defining and predicting tracheoesophageal puncture success. Arch Otolaryngol Head Neck Surg. 1992;118(8):811–6. https://doi.org/10.1001/archotol.1992.01880080033009.
10. Sylvester MJ, Marchiano E, Park RC, Baredes S, Eloy JA. Impact of chronic obstructive pulmonary disease on patients undergoing laryngectomy for laryngeal cancer. Laryngoscope. 2017;127(2):417–23. https://doi.org/10.1002/lary.26050. Epub 2016 May 30.

11. Longobardi Y, Savoia V, Bussu F, Morra L, Mari G, Nesci DA, Parrilla C, D'Alatri L. Integrated rehabilitation after total laryngectomy: a pilot trial study. Support Care Cancer. 2019;27(9):3537–44. https://doi.org/10.1007/s00520-019-4647-1. Epub 2019 Jan 26.
12. Singer S, Meyer A, Fuchs M, Schock J, Pabst F, Vogel HJ, Oeken J, Sandner A, Koscielny S, Hormes K, Breitenstein K, Dietz A. Motivation as a predictor of speech intelligibility after total laryngectomy. Head Neck. 2013;35(6):836–46. https://doi.org/10.1002/hed.23043. Epub 2012 Jun 25.
13. Huang SH, O'Sullivan B. Overview of the 8th edition TNM classification for head and neck cancer. Curr Treat Options Oncol. 2017;18(7):40. https://doi.org/10.1007/s11864-017-0484-y.
14. Chakravarty PD, McMurran AEL, Banigo A, Shakeel M, Ah-See KW. Primary versus secondary tracheoesophageal puncture: systematic review and meta-analysis. J Laryngol Otol. 2018;132(1):14–21. https://doi.org/10.1017/S0022215117002390. Epub 2017 Nov 27.
15. Barauna Neto JC, Dedivitis RA, Aires FT, Pfann RZ, Matos LL, Cernea CR. Comparison between primary and secondary tracheoesophageal puncture prosthesis: a systematic review. ORL J Otorhinolaryngol Relat Spec. 2017;79(4):222–9. https://doi.org/10.1159/000477970. Epub 2017 Jul 29.
16. Panwar A, Militsakh O, Lindau R, Coughlin A, Sayles H, Rieke KR, Lydiatt W, Lydiatt D, Smith R. Impact of primary tracheoesophageal puncture on outcomes after total laryngectomy. Otolaryngol Head Neck Surg. 2018;158(1):103–9. https://doi.org/10.1177/0194599817722938. Epub 2017 Aug 15.
17. Singer MI, Blom ED. An endoscopic technique for restoration of voice after laryngectomy. Ann Otol Rhinol Laryngol. 1980;89(6 Pt 1):529–33. https://doi.org/10.1177/000348948008900608.
18. Scherl C, Kauffels J, Schützenberger A, Döllinger M, Bohr C, Dürr S, Fietkau R, Haderlein M, Koch M, Traxdorf M, Mantsopoulos K, Müller S, Iro H. Secondary tracheoesophageal puncture after laryngectomy increases complications with shunt and voice prosthesis. Laryngoscope. 2020;130(12):E865–73. https://doi.org/10.1002/lary.28517. Epub 2020 Feb 6.
19. Luu K, Chang BA, Valenzuela D, Anderson D. Primary versus secondary tracheoesophageal puncture for voice rehabilitation in laryngectomy patients: a systematic review. Clin Otolaryngol. 2018;43(5):1250–9. https://doi.org/10.1111/coa.13138. Epub 2018 May 31.
20. Sinclair CF, Rosenthal EL, McColloch NL, Magnuson JS, Desmond RA, Peters GE, Carroll WR. Primary versus delayed tracheoesophageal puncture for laryngopharyngectomy with free flap reconstruction. Laryngoscope. 2011;121(7):1436–40. https://doi.org/10.1002/lary.21836. Epub 2011 May 3.
21. Boscolo-Rizzo P, Zanetti F, Carpené S, Da Mosto MC. Long-term results with tracheoesophageal voice prosthesis: primary versus secondary TEP. Eur Arch Otorrinolaringol. 2008;265(1):73–7. https://doi.org/10.1007/s00405-007-0423-9. Epub 2007 Aug 23.
22. Sayles M, Grant DG. Preventing pharyngo-cutaneous fistula in total laryngectomy: a systematic review and meta-analysis. Laryngoscope. 2014;124(5):1150–63. https://doi.org/10.1002/lary.24448. Epub 2013 Nov 15.
23. Emerick KS, Tomycz L, Bradford CR, Lyden TH, Chepeha DB, Wolf GT, Teknos TN. Primary versus secondary tracheoesophageal puncture in salvage total laryngectomy following chemoradiation. Otolaryngol Head Neck Surg. 2009;140(3):386–90. https://doi.org/10.1016/j.otohns.2008.10.018.

Surgical Techniques

3

3.1 Primary Tracheoesophageal Puncture

Primary TEP consists in the creation of a tracheoesophageal fistula with VP placement at the end of total laryngectomy surgery. However, some precautions of surgical technique should be carried out in order to ensure optimal functioning and easy care of the TEP.

3.1.1 Section of Trachea/Trachea Dissection

The section of the trachea should be performed including at least 2–3 tracheal rings, below the cricoid, in relation to the height of the upper esophageal sphincter (UES). Indeed, the TEP should be performed below the so-called *pharyngo-esophageal segment (PES)*, namely the section of esophagus that allow us to make sound (Fig. 3.1).

The most used trachea section techniques are circle, flute spout (or bevel), and triangular [1]. In our opinion, the circle technique is the best since the integrity of the cartilaginous tracheal ring ensures greater stability of the tracheostoma and reduces the incidence of tracheostomal stenosis. In fact, in our opinion, the interruption of the integrity of the tracheal ring leads to loss of circumferential rigidity. Moreover, the size of the tracheostoma is important too. Indeed, it must be large enough to allow breathing without the need for a tracheal tube but small enough to ensure its easy occlusion for phonation [2].

Supplementary Information The online version contains supplementary material available at https://doi.org/10.1007/978-3-031-29654-3_3. The videos can be accessed individually by clicking the DOI link in the accompanying figure caption or by scanning this link with the SN More Media App.

3.1.2 Neurotomy of Monolateral Pharyngeal Plexus and/or Monolateral Cricopharyngeal Muscle Myotomy

These two surgical procedures are usually performed to avoid a possible complication in laryngectomized patients with speech prosthesis: pharyngeal hypertonicity with consequent phonatory and swallowing troubles (Figs. 3.2, 3.3, 3.4, 3.5).

In 1986, Singer et al. reported an increased risk of pharyngocutaneous fistula (PCF) after pharyngeal myotomy due to reduced vascularization of the hypopharynx [3]. For this reason, they had introduced and studied another technique: the neurotomy of the pharyngeal plexus. This procedure was more advantageous because it did not impair the pharyngeal vascularization and ensures a residual tension of the pharyngo-esophageal segment too. Based on these observations, in 1995, Blom et al. deepened this topic dividing the examined population (laryngectomized patients with primary TEP) into three groups according to the technique performed: (1) neurotomy, (2) myotomy, and (3) neurotomy plus myotomy [4]. These three groups were analyzed 12 months after surgery in terms of change of developing

Fig. 3.1 Pharyngoesophageal segment (PES)

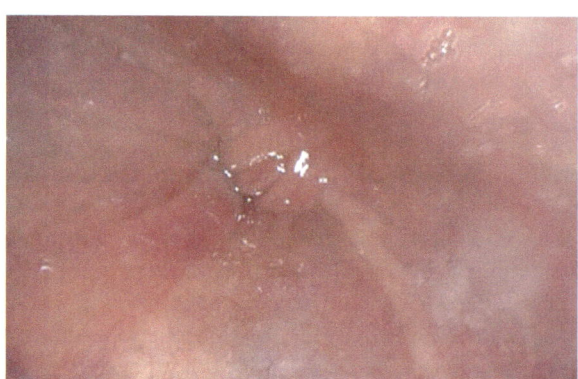

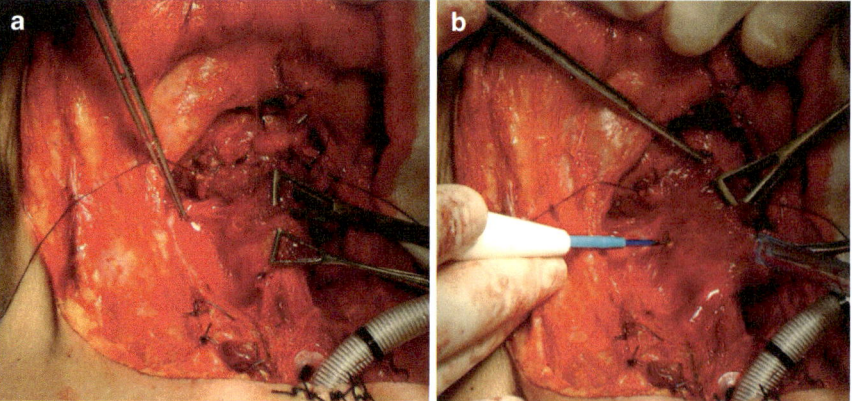

Fig. 3.2 Right pharyngeal plexus (**a**); neurotomy of right pharyngeal plexus (**b**)

Fig. 3.3 Neurotomy of pharyngeal plexus

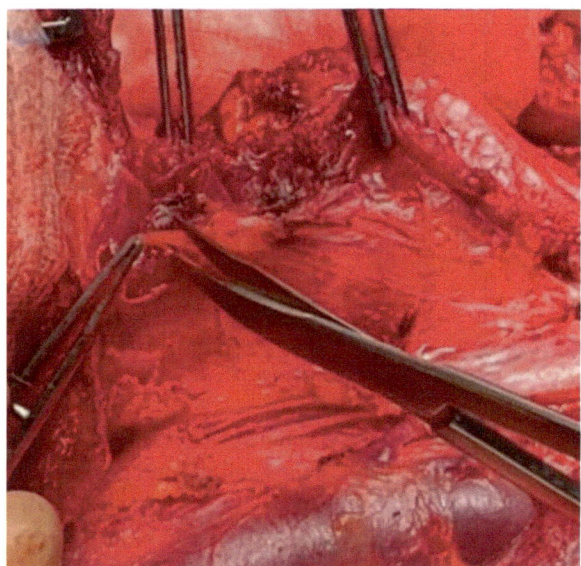

Fig. 3.4 Monolateral cricopharyngeal muscle myotomy

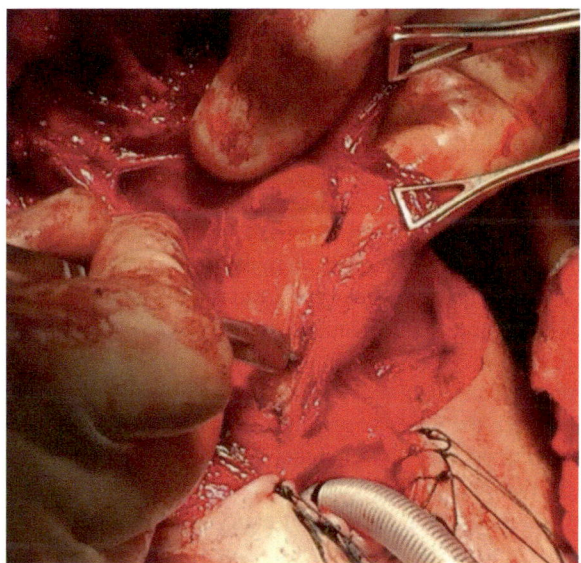

pharyngospasm and in terms of phonatory outcome (maximum phonation time and fundamental frequency). As regard to the prevention of pharyngeal hypertonicity, the study showed that the three techniques had the same results. As regard to the phonatory result, the study showed that: (a) the only neurotomy provided a higher fundamental frequency thanks to the compensation of the contralateral pharyngeal plexus that ensures minimal tension of the pharynx; (b) the maximum phonation

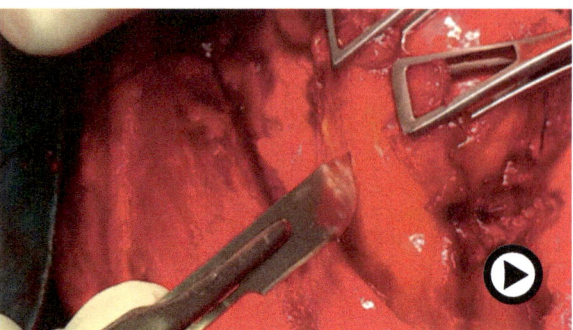

Fig. 3.5 Monolateral cricopharyngeal muscle myotomy (▶ https://doi.org/10.1007/000-bmn)

time is achieved in the combined neurotomy and myotomy surgery as it guarantees both the compensation of the healthy contralateral pharyngeal plexus and the hypotonia of the pharynx due to myotomy, as previously written.

3.1.3   Pharyngeal Suture

The suture of the pharynx can be performed in different ways: a tobacco bag with a single suture thread, vertically or horizontally oriented suture or "T-shaped" suture. This surgical step is important and critical for the success of the surgery since a suture that is not properly performed is related to high risk of PCF, common complication in patients undergoing total laryngectomy [5–7].

The effectiveness of the pharyngeal suture is based on two parameters: the suture line and the suture technique [8]. In particular, the tobacco bag closure was designed by Portmann and consists in making a bag of tobacco around the pharyngostoma, by folding mucosal edges back inside. The vertical or horizontal line sutures consist of a continuous or interrupted suture, vertically or horizontally oriented, respectively. In our opinion, the T-shaped suture ensures the greatest tightness and resistance to the tension; in this case, the horizontal branch of the suture corresponds to the suture between the pharynx and the lingual base (Fig. 3.6). However, this technique has a weakness: the point of suture where the three structures converge (tongue base and the two pharyngeal flaps) [9].

In addition to the type of pharyngeal closure, the suture technique may also be different: non-piercing/drilling or folding mucosa back inside, extra-mucosa on constrictor muscle fascia, continuous or interrupted suture (Connell technique) [8]. In this regard, a 2015 study compared the technique of interrupted suture and the technique of continuous suture, proving that the latter statistically significant correlates with a lower risk of developing PCF [10]. Relatively recent is the mechanical suture by linear stapler [11] that has many advantages over manual suturing: pharyngeal closure is waterproof, no tension at the suture level, no opening of the pharynx resulting in minimal risk of contamination of the surgical field, better hemostasis [12]. However, the use of the stapler for the pharyngeal closure

Fig. 3.6 T-shaped suture
of pharynx

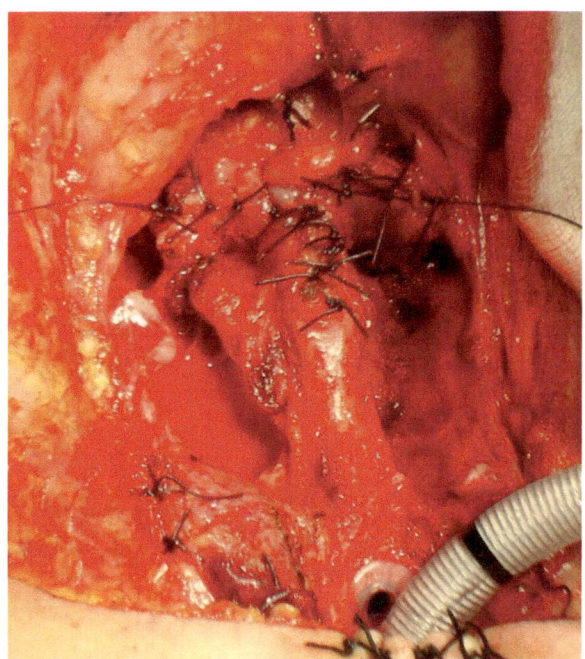

is closely dependent on the site and extension of laryngeal cancer. Indeed, the surgical stapler can only be used for intralaryngeal tumors with anterior extension in order to ensure the oncological radicality since the use of this device makes it more difficult to assess the extension of cancer, especially if it is marginal. Moreover, collecting frozen sections or mucosal samples as free margin is difficult or even impossible [13].

3.1.4   Flattening and Stability of Tracheostoma

In order to ensure a stable tracheostoma over time to allow proper functioning and easy replacement of the voice prosthesis, it is recommended not only to maintain the size of the trachea, by preserving the integrity of cartilaginous ring, but also to suture this ring to the lower cervical skin flap for almost all of its circumference [2] taking care to cover the tracheal ring with the skin to avoid complications such as infections, perichondritis, and stenosis [14] (Figs. 3.7 and 3.8). Indeed, disruption of cartilaginous ring, as required in primary suture techniques or in some surgical techniques for enlargement plastic of tracheostoma (oblique, triangular) [1], exposes the risk of tracheostomal stenosis or its recurrence.

Moreover, it is important to keep in mind that a tracheostoma can change over time its position and width: it can be stretched down and thus it can become a deep stoma, while maintaining its width, or it may be subject to shrinkage (Fig. 3.9).

Fig. 3.7 Suture of the tracheal ring to the lower cervical skin flap for almost all of its circumference

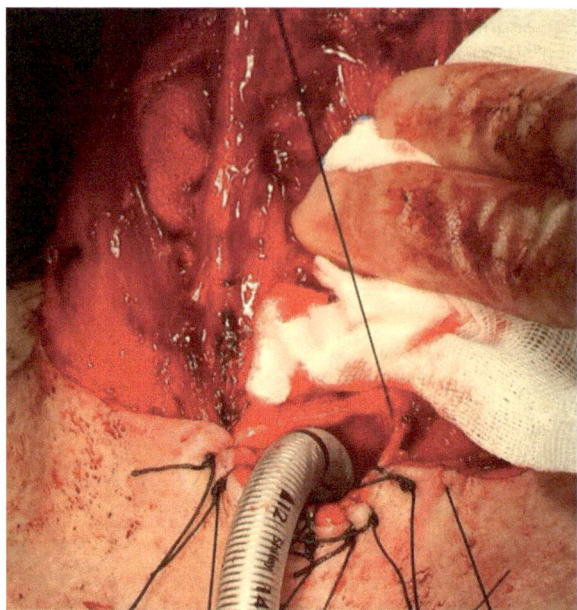

Fig. 3.8 Suture of the tracheal ring to the lower cervical skin flap for almost all of its circumference

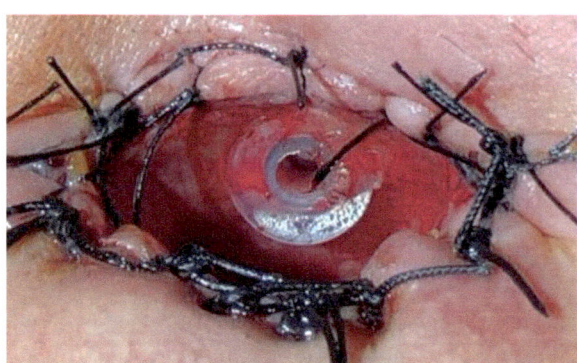

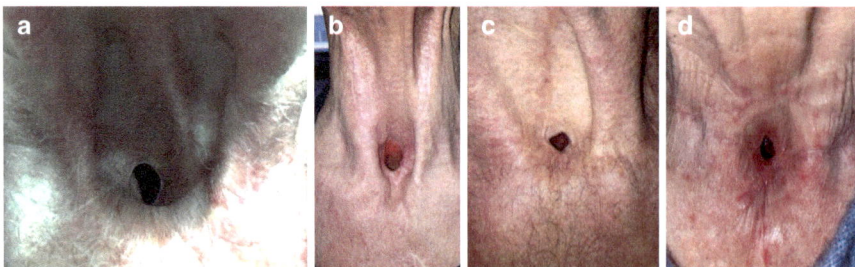

Fig. 3.9 Deep stoma (**a**, **b**) and stomal stenosis (**c**, **d**)

Fig. 3.10 Desirable tracheostoma: proper width and stability of the tracheostoma thanks to muscle support

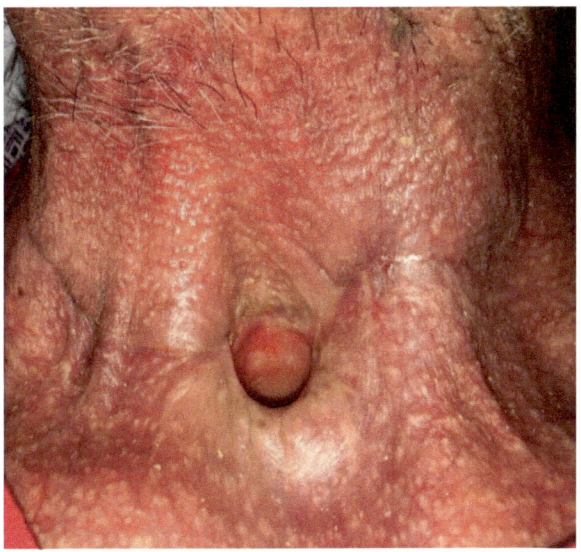

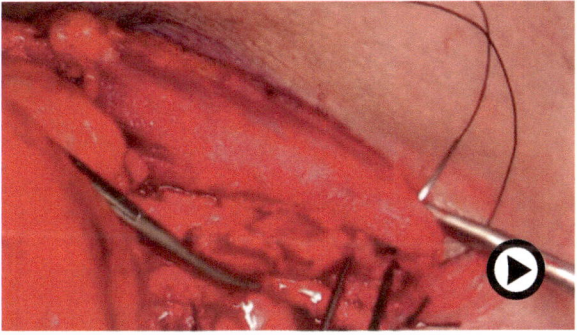

Fig. 3.11 Suture between lower cervical skin flap, sternocleidomastoid muscle, and tracheal ring (▶ https://doi.org/10.1007/000-bmk)

Therefore, the goal is to achieve a tracheostoma of optimal size and placed on the same level of skin in order to allow its easy occlusion and phonation with VP (Fig. 3.10).

For this purpose, the edge of the sternal head of the sternocleidomastoid muscle (SCM) may be cut in order to ensure the flattening of the stoma, depending on the surgical techniques [2, 15] or it can be sutured and attached to the lateral wall of the trachea (Fig. 3.11).

This measure can guarantee both an adequate width of the tracheostoma and its greater stability over time thanks to muscle support (Fig. 3.12). When choosing the best strategy, the patient's cervical anatomical characteristics should be taken into account. Indeed, in case of a lean neck, the protection of the jugular by the dissected sternal head of the SCM muscle would be missing resulting in vein placement just under the skin (Fig. 3.13).

Fig. 3.12 Desirable
tracheostoma: optimal size
and placed on the same
level of skin

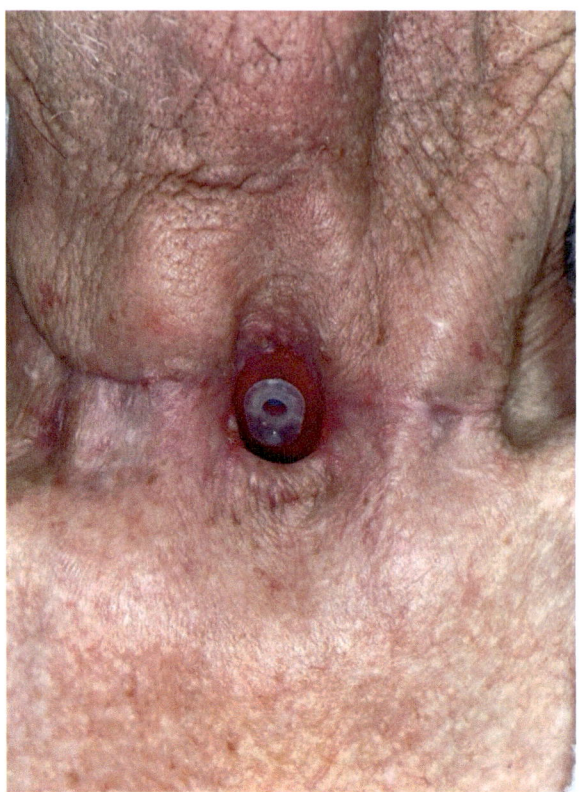

Fig. 3.13 Axial CT scan:
sternocleidomastoid
muscle (SCM) covers
internal jugular vein (IJV)

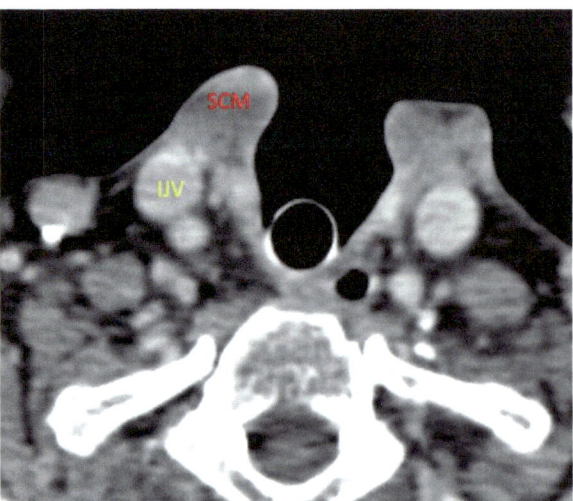

3.1.5   Techniques for the TEP and Voice Prosthesis Placement

The techniques for TEP creation are comparable between the two types of prostheses most often used (Provox®, Blom-Singer®): indeed, they both require a pharyngeal protector and a trocar. In particular, the Provox® voice prosthesis has a retrograde positioning mode (from the inside to the outside) (Fig. 3.14): once the tracheoesophageal fistula is made, the VP is introduced from the esophageal side to the tracheal side, through a progressive dilator.

Conversely, the Blom-Singer® VP has an anterograde positioning mode (from the outside to the inside): placed inside a progressive dilator, the VP passes through the tracheaesophageal wall (Figs. 3.15 and 3.16).

As first placement, a prosthesis 10–12 mm long is usually used, chosen according to the thickness of the tracheoesophageal wall evaluated with an appropriate

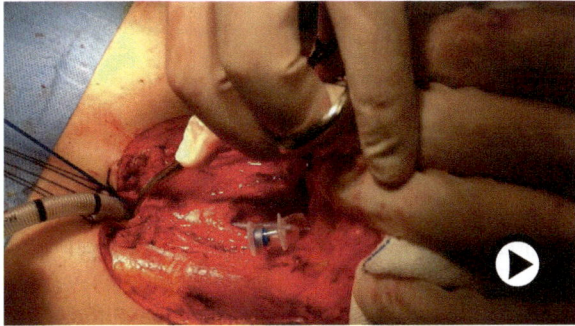

Fig. 3.14   Primary TEP with Provox® voice prosthesis (▶ https://doi.org/10.1007/000-bmm)

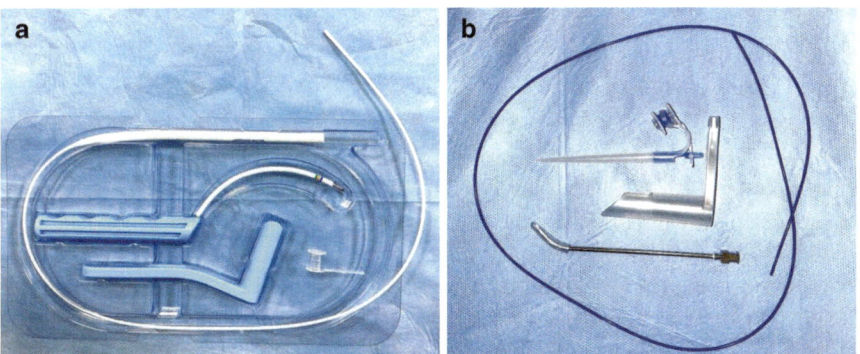

Fig. 3.15   Blom-Singer® (**a**) and Provox® (**b**) kit for primary TEP

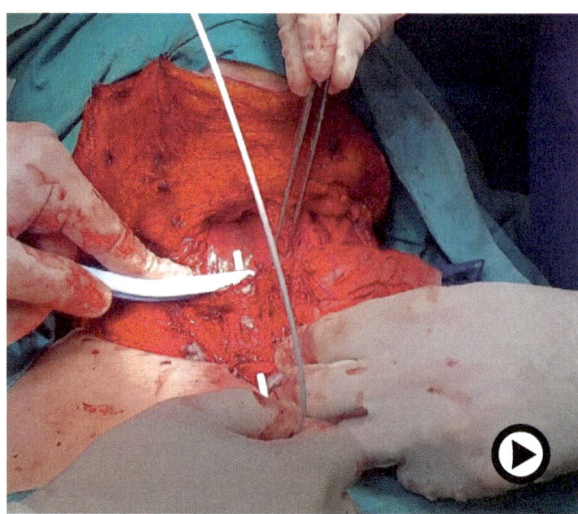

Fig. 3.16 Primary TEP with Blom-Singer® voice prosthesis (▶ https://doi.org/10.1007/000-bmj)

meter, always considering the inevitable post-operative edema which causes a momentary increase [16]. The width of the prosthesis usually has a diameter of 16 Fr or 20 Fr so as to ensure easy vocal emission in post-op. A 2016 study compared 16 Fr and 20 Fr initial vocal prosthesis in terms of risk of developing complications and voice outcome. The study showed that there was no statistically significant difference between the two diameters of VP in terms of complications; however, the study advised the use of 16 Fr VP for two main reasons: less tissue trauma during execution of TEP and the possibility to place the 20 Fr VP in case of an enlarged fistula without the need for much wider prostheses (22 Fr) or a custom-made prosthesis [17].

3.2   Secondary TEP

Secondary TEP consists in the positioning of the voice prosthesis after a distance of time from total laryngectomy surgery. The measures described in the primary technique are equally important for the successful creation of TEP with secondary technique. Indeed, if during the total laryngectomy, these precautions have been carried out, no pre-operative evaluation is required to assess the PES functionality and the height where the puncture should be performed: original or revisited Taub test (Fig. 3.17) [18]. However, the Taub test is burdened with a risk of false positivity between 10 and 30% [18, 19].

The most widely used technique for secondary TEP involves the use of a rigid esophagoscope that allows the protection of the posterior wall of the esophagus and the structures underlying it from the introduction of the trocar, whatever the prosthesis to be placed (Figs. 3.18 and 3.19).

Fig. 3.17 Taub test

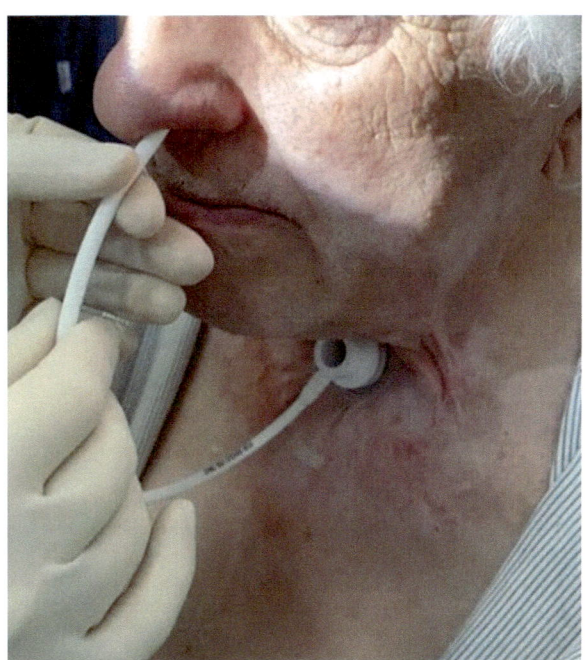

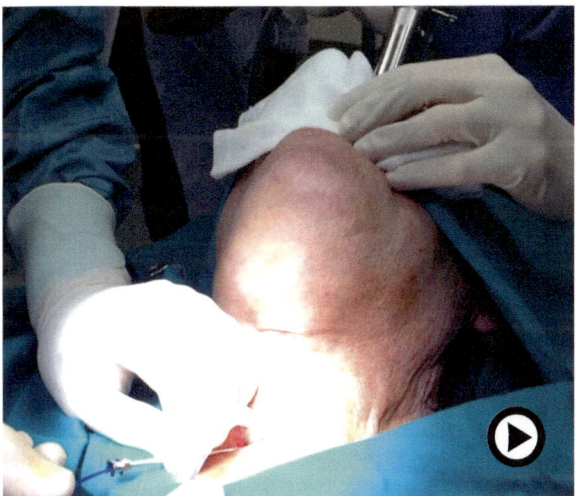

Fig. 3.18 Secondary TEP using rigid esophagoscope and Provox® insertion kit (▶ https://doi.org/10.1007/000-bmp)

Therefore, this technique is necessarily performed under general anesthesia. However, in some cases, the use of the rigid esophagoscope may be difficult or impossible due to several reasons such as pharyngeal stenosis, pharyngeal reconstructions with flap, stiffness of the cervical spine, limited mouth opening, etc. In

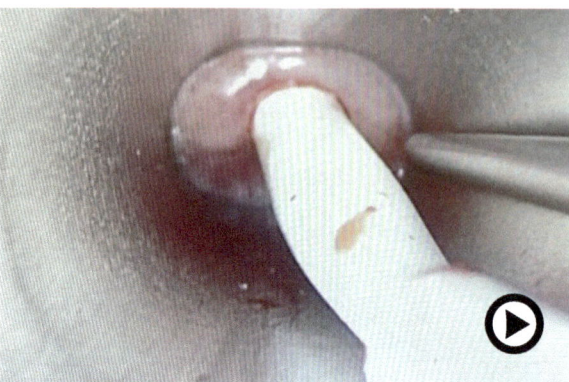

Fig. 3.19 Secondary TEP using rigid esophagoscope and Blom-Singer® insertion kit (vision from inside) (▶ https://doi.org/10.1007/000-bmq)

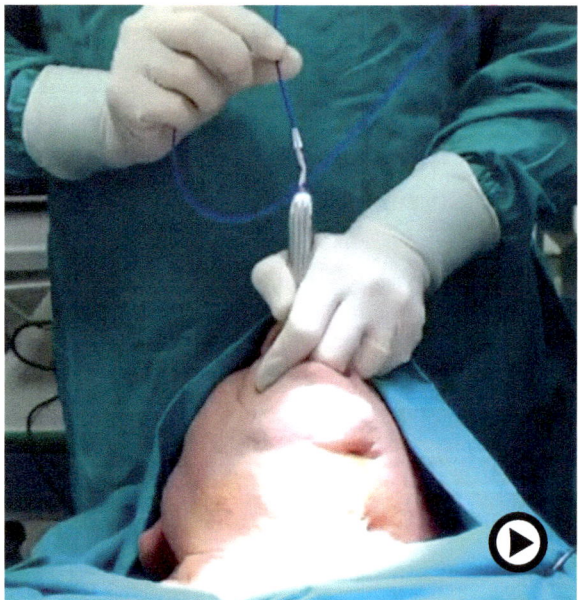

Fig. 3.20 Secondary TEP using Yankauer suction tube and Provox® insertion kit (▶ https://doi.org/10.1007/000-bmr)

such situations, the so-called blind techniques are performed by using tools that allow to reach the correct site of placement of the prosthesis safely: hysterometer [20], Yankauer suction tube, esophagoscope with working channel, and endotracheal tube [21] (Fig. 3.20).

In this regard, in 2013, Fukuhara et al. proposed a new secondary TEP technique—further amended by Hanai et al. [22]—which involves the use of flexible rhinolaryngoscope with a working channel and a biopsy needle [23]. This technique has two main advantages: it can be performed on an outpatient basis under local anesthesia and consists of an "inside out TEP," so the tracheoesophageal puncture is created from the inside (esophageal lumen) to the outside (tracheal lumen). This technique gives maximum safety because it is performed under endoscopic vision and because it avoids damaging the posterior wall of the esophagus (with risk of mediastinitis). However, patient compliance in performing this procedure—that still remains invasive—in outpatient and under local anesthesia should always be considered.

3.2.1 Complications of the Secondary TEP

Secondary TEP may lead to major and minor complications. The latter correspond to the complications of an endoscopy of the upper airways: Trauma to the lips and/or teeth, mucosal lacerations, bleeding due to vessel injury of flap used for pharyngeal reconstruction.

The major complications are mainly related to the use of the rigid esophagoscope. Indeed, a tortuous or stenotic pharynx or a deformity of the cervical spine may make the placement of the rigid esophagoscope technically difficult exposing the patient to complications such as perforation of the esophagus resulting in mediastinitis, fracture or infection of the cervical spine, and cervical osteomyelitis [24].

Therefore, since the major complications are prerogative of the secondary TEP technique, primary TEP should be considered the first choice in most cases.

Declaration by Authors   Figures are original and free from copyright issues.

References

1. Suzuki M, Tsunoda A, Shirakura S, Sumi T, Nishijima W, Kishimoto S. A novel permanent tracheostomy technique for prevention of stomal stenosis (triangular tracheostomy). Auris Nasus Larynx. 2010;37(4):465–8. https://doi.org/10.1016/j.anl.2009.11.007. Epub 2009 Dec 29.
2. Verschuur HP, Gregor RT, Hilgers FJ, Balm AJ. The tracheostoma in relation to prosthetic voice rehabilitation. Laryngoscope. 1996;106(1 Pt 1):111–5. https://doi.org/10.1097/00005537-199601000-00022.
3. Singer MI, Blom ED, Hamaker RC. Pharyngeal plexus neurectomy for alaryngeal speech rehabilitation. Laryngoscope. 1986;96(1):50–4. https://doi.org/10.1288/00005537-198601000-00008.
4. Blom ED, Pauloski BR, Hamaker RC. Functional outcome after surgery for prevention of pharyngospasms in tracheoesophageal speakers. Part I: Speech characteristics. Laryngoscope. 1995;105(10):1093–103. https://doi.org/10.1288/00005537-199510000-00016.
5. Park J, Chang C, Kwon D. Use of fibrin adhesive for preventing pharyngocutaneous fistula in total laryngectomy. Am J Otolaryngol. 2020;41(6):102674. https://doi.org/10.1016/j.amjoto.2020.102674. Epub 2020 Aug 13.
6. Higashino T, Oshima A, Fukunaga Y, Hayashi R. Surgical outcome of pharyngocutaneous fistula after total laryngectomy: a retrospective study. Ann Plast Surg. 2021;87(4):431–4. https://doi.org/10.1097/SAP.0000000000002769.
7. Massaro N, Verro B, Greco G, Chianetta E, D'Ecclesia A, Saraniti C. Quality of life with voice prosthesis after total laryngectomy. Iran J Otorhinolaryngol. 2021;33(118):301–9. https://doi.org/10.22038/ijorl.2021.53724.2832. PMID: 34692577; PMCID: PMC8507945.

8. Avci H, Karabulut B. Is it important which suturing technique used for pharyngeal muco-sal closure in total laryngectomy? Modified continuous Connell suture may decrease pharyngocutaneous fistula. Ear Nose Throat J. 2020;99(10):664–70. https://doi.org/10.1177/0145561320938918. Epub 2020 Jul 23.
9. Singer MI, Blom ED. Selective myotomy for voice restoration after total laryngectomy. Arch Otolaryngol. 1981;107(11):670–3. https://doi.org/10.1001/archotol.1981.00790470018005.
10. Deniz M, Ciftci Z, Gultekin E. Pharyngoesophageal suturing technique may decrease the incidence of pharyngocutaneous fistula following total laryngectomy. Surg Res Pract. 2015;2015:363640. https://doi.org/10.1155/2015/363640. Epub 2015 Aug 5. PMID: 26366434; PMCID: PMC4541018.
11. Bedrin L, Ginsburg G, Horowitz Z, Talmi YP. 25-Year experience of using a linear stapler in laryngectomy. Head Neck. 2005;27(12):1073–9. https://doi.org/10.1002/hed.20280.
12. Gonçalves AJ, de Souza JA Jr, Menezes MB, Kavabata NK, Suehara AB, Lehn CN. Pharyngocutaneous fistulae following total laryngectomy comparison between man-ual and mechanical sutures. Eur Arch Otorrinolaringol. 2009;266(11):1793–8. https://doi.org/10.1007/s00405-009-0945-4. Epub 2009 Mar 13.
13. Chiesa-Estomba CM, Mayo-Yanez M, Palacios-García JM, Lechien JR, Viljoen G, Karkos PD, Barillari MR, González-García JA, Sistiaga-Suarez JA, González-Botas JH, Ayad T, Ferlito A. Stapler-assisted pharyngeal closure after total laryngectomy: a systematic review and meta-analysis. Oncol Ther. 2022;10(1):241–52. https://doi.org/10.1007/s40487-022-00193-5. Epub 2022 Mar 31. PMID: 35357676; PMCID: PMC9098751.
14. Lorenz KJ, Maier H. Pulmonale Rehabilitation nach totaler Laryngektomie durch die Verwendung von HME (Heat Moisture Exchanger) [Pulmonary rehabilitation after total laryngectomy using a heat and moisture exchanger (HME)]. Laryngorhinootologie. 2009;88(8):513–22. https://doi.org/10.1055/s-0029-1225619. Epub 2009 Jul 30.
15. Santoro GP, Luparello P, Lazio MS, Comini LV, Martelli F, Cannavicci A. Myotomy of ster-nocleidomastoid muscle as a secondary procedure in laryngectomized patients. Head Neck. 2019;41(10):3743–6. https://doi.org/10.1002/hed.25852. Epub 2019 Jul 26.
16. Lundy DS, Landera MA, Bremekamp J, Weed D. Longitudinal tracheoesophageal puncture size stability. Otolaryngol Head Neck Surg. 2012;147(5):885–8. https://doi.org/10.1177/0194599812449293. Epub 2012 May 22.
17. Naunheim MR, Remenschneider AK, Scangas GA, Bunting GW, Deschler DG. The effect of initial tracheoesophageal voice prosthesis size on postoperative complica-tions and voice outcomes. Ann Otol Rhinol Laryngol. 2016;125(6):478–84. https://doi.org/10.1177/0003489415620426. Epub 2015 Dec 9.
18. Sirin AA, Erdim I, Baykal B, Oghan F, Yilmazer R, Guvey A, Kayhan FT. Detection of ideal reservoir level after laryngectomy using endoilluminator in voice rehabilitation. Laryngoscope. 2015;125(7):E239–44. https://doi.org/10.1002/lary.25213. Epub 2015 Feb 20.
19. Sloane PM, Griffin JF, O'Dwyer TP. Esophageal insufflation and videofluoroscopy for evaluation of esophageal speech in laryngectomy patients: clinical implications (Erratum in: Radiology 1992 Mar;182(3):899. Griffin JM [corrected to Griffin JF].). Radiology. 1991;181(2):433–7. https://doi.org/10.1148/radiology.181.2.1924785.
20. Gazzini L, Laura E, Molteni G, Marchioni D, Pighi GP. Secondary tracheoesopha-geal puncture with the blind technique: 10 years' experience. Eur Arch Otorrinolaringol. 2021;278(11):4459–67. https://doi.org/10.1007/s00405-021-06674-z. Epub 2021 Feb 13.
21. Abdul-Aziz D, Zenga J, Deschler DG. The difficult secondary tracheoesophageal puncture: a technique for safe insertion. ORL J Otorhinolaryngol Relat Spec. 2019;81(1):10–5. https://doi.org/10.1159/000492968. Epub 2018 Nov 28.
22. Hanai N, Beppu S, Nishikawa D, Terada H, Nishikawa D, Sawabe M. A novel procedure of secondary voice prosthesis insertion from the inside out: the modified Fukuhara method. Auris Nasus Larynx. 2022;49(4):658–62. https://doi.org/10.1016/j.anl.2021.11.006. Epub 2021 Dec 4.

23. Fukuhara T, Fujiwara K, Nomura K, Miyake N, Kitano H. New method for in-office secondary voice prosthesis insertion under local anesthesia by reverse puncture from esophageal lumen. Ann Otol Rhinol Laryngol. 2013;122(3):163–8. https://doi.org/10.1177/000348941312200304.
24. Malik T, Bruce I, Cherry J. Surgical complications of tracheo-oesophageal puncture and speech valves. Curr Opin Otolaryngol Head Neck Surg. 2007;15(2):117–22. https://doi.org/10.1097/MOO.0b013e3280964dc8.

Complications

4

4.1 Background

Complications can be divided into two main categories: (1) related to tracheoesophageal puncture (TEP), (2) related to voice prosthesis (VP) [1].

Studies have shown that many complications are due to improper management of VP and TEP by the patient, emphasizing the importance of providing correct information and education to patients about the management of the prosthesis [2]. Moreover, patients should be warned and trained about the so-called red flags, meaning the predictive signs of possible complications. Indeed, if the patient is well trained, it is possible to take action early avoiding complications that would require more invasive remedial measures.

The current literature agrees that there is no greater rate of complications after radiation therapy (RT) [1, 3]. In particular, Scherl et al. claim that adjuvant RT is not related with increased risk of complications, rather the creation of TEP with VP placement after radiation therapy can lead to the onset of complications. For this reason, the authors recommend the creation of the TEP concurrently with the total laryngectomy or before starting the RT [3].

4.2 Complications Related to TEP

One of the most frequent TEP complications is peri-prosthetic leakage (or leakage around the VP) that occurs in more than 70% of laryngectomy patients [4]. Moreover, the peri-prosthetic leakage should be considered more correctly as a consequence of

---

Supplementary Information The online version contains supplementary material available at https://doi.org/10.1007/978-3-031-29654-3_4. The videos can be accessed individually by clicking the DOI link in the accompanying figure caption or by scanning this link with the SN More Media App.

other complications such as fistula enlargement, presence of granulation tissue, and peri-fistula inflammation [3].

4.2.1 Enlargement of the TEP

The TEP may increase in diameter resulting in leakage of saliva and/or food in the trachea around the VP. The main causes are two: (1) atrophy of peri-prosthetic tissues with thinning of the esophageal–tracheal wall which usually occurs after years with minimal tendency to spontaneous shrinkage (Fig. 4.1); (2) the phlogistic–necrotic processes that may occur due to too short prosthesis that applies excessive pressure on the esophageal mucosa or due to repeated trauma from digital occlusion of the stoma during phonation [5]. In this case, Lundy et al. have reported that about 90% of patients undergo a TEP size modification with need to change the length or diameter of the VP within the first 3 years [6].

There are several solutions to overcome this complication: silicon ring, prosthesis with an extra, enlarged esophageal flange, prosthesis with larger esophageal and tracheal flanges [7, 8] (Fig. 4.2), purse-string suture around fistula [9], collagen injection [10], vox implant, fibrin glue, and autologous fat [11, 12]. In this regard, the algorithm for the management of peri-prosthetic leakage proposed by Parilla et al. [13] proves to be very valuable (Fig. 4.3).

Another risk factor for peri-prosthetic leakage due to widened TEP is the gastro-esophageal reflux disease (GERD), which is quite frequent in patients undergoing total laryngectomy. Zhang et al. have observed a prevalence close to 50% of minor peristaltic alterations and a prevalence of about 30% of major disorders of peristalsis after total laryngectomy [14]. Although to date the pathogenesis is unknown, total laryngectomy surgery involves hypopharyngeal and esophageal functional and morphological changes resulting in impaired esophageal motility. One of the consequences of esophageal dysmotility is gastro-esophageal reflux that occurs

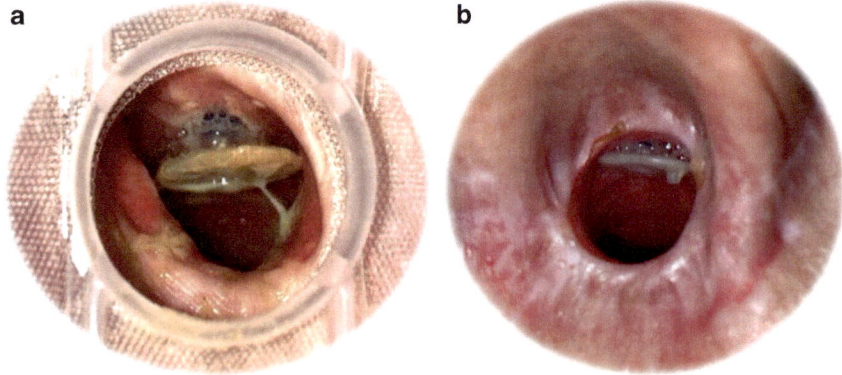

Fig. 4.1 Peri-prosthetic leakage due to bad management (**a**) and due to thinned tracheoesophageal wall (**b**)

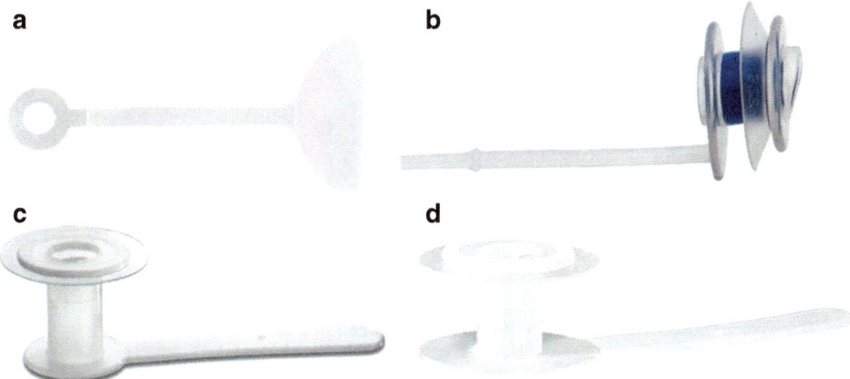

Fig. 4.2 Silicon ring (**a**), prosthesis with an extra enlarged esophageal flange (**b**), prosthesis with large esophageal flange (**c**), prosthesis with large esophageal and tracheal flanges (**d**)

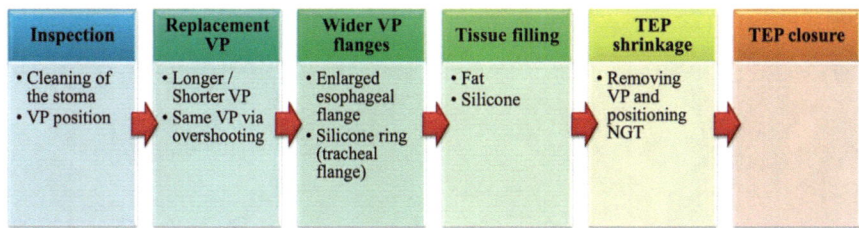

Fig. 4.3 Management of peri-prosthetic leakage. *VP* voice prosthesis, *TEP* tracheoesophageal puncture, *NGT* nasogastric tube. [Based on Parrilla C, Longobardi Y, Galli J, Rigante M, Paludetti G, Bussu F, Scarano E. Periprosthetic Leakage in Tracheoesophageal Prosthesis: Proposal of a Standardized Therapeutic Algorithm. Otolaryngol Head Neck Surg. 2021 Sep;165(3):446–454. doi: 10.1177/0194599820983343]

with high incidence in laryngectomy patients. Danic Hadzibegovic et al. have demonstrated that gastro-esophageal reflux can cause peri-prosthetic leakage due to atrophy with consequent enlargement of the fistula and the onset of peri-prosthetic tracheal granulations. Based on this finding, the authors suggested daily therapy with proton pump inhibitor (PPI), proving its effectiveness of prolonging the average life of the prosthesis and in reducing damage to peri-prosthetic tissues and therefore the risk of voice prosthesis complications [15].

Caution Using larger diameter, VP is not recommended because it could cause a further increase in its TEP size, if the enlargement of the TEP is due to laxity of adjacent tissues.

The most fearsome complication of a fistula too wide is dislocation with loss of the VP. This can occur posteriorly in the esophagus (Fig. 4.4) with transit of the prosthesis to the digestive tract (Fig. 4.5) and his expulsion with feces, although rare

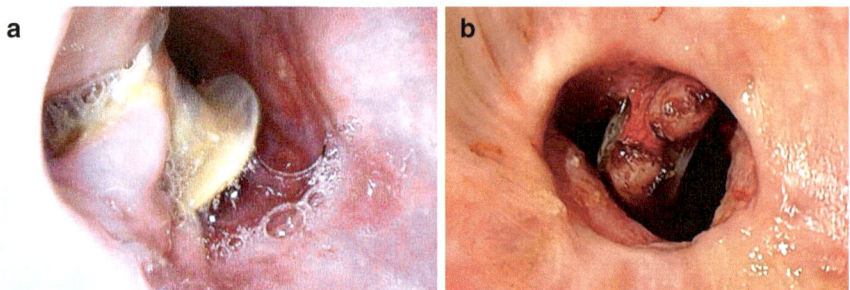

Fig. 4.4   Voice prosthesis dislocation in esophagus (**a**) and in trachea (**b**)

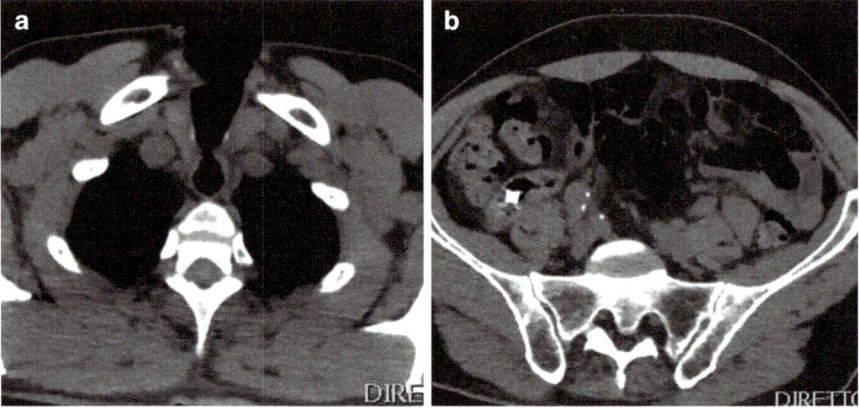

Fig. 4.5   Empty tracheoesophageal fistula (**a**), voice prosthesis in the bowel (**b**)

episodes of intestinal occlusion at the ileocecal valve level have been described [16]. Otherwise, the voice prosthesis can fall anteriorly into the trachea and can obstruct a bronchus resulting in severe dyspnea: this incident represents an emergency.

4.2.2   TEP Tract Hypertrophy/Stricture

Peri-prosthetic hyperemia and edema may indicate the presence of an infection (Fig. 4.6).

Depending on the articles, this occurs in about 30% of patients [4]. In these cases, oral antibiotic and steroidal therapy and the placement of a silicon ring to reduce the risk of peri-prosthetic leakage are recommended. Once fixed the acute event, the voice prosthesis is replaced if it is damaged or colonized by bacteria or fungi.

It should be noted that hypertrophic tissue may involve VP extrusion or displacement; in other cases, the mucosal redundancy may cover the whole prosthesis. In

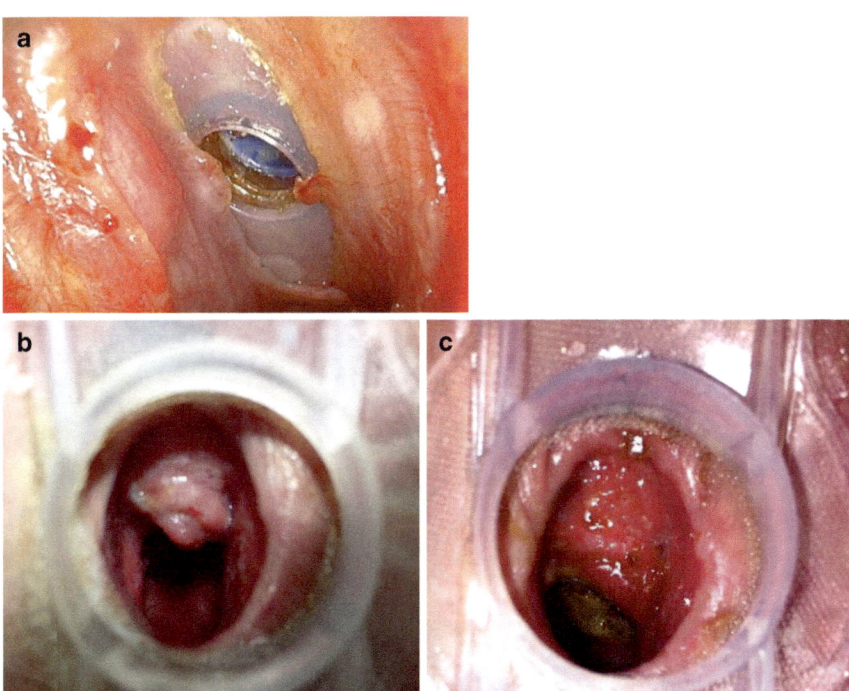

Fig. 4.6 Peri-prosthetic hyperemia and phlogosis (**a, b**), tracheoesophageal puncture hypertrophy (**c**)

some cases, these patients have previously undergone surgery for widening the stenotic tracheostoma. Indeed, during surgery, only the tracheal stenotic ring is removed without affecting the back wall of the trachea, where the TEP is found. The posterior wall of the trachea unaffected from surgery results higher than the upper edge of the tracheostoma and no longer tightened by the tracheal ring. Therefore, this tracheal mucosa tends to fold in on itself, resulting redundant (Fig. 4.7).

Rarely, TEP may undergo stenosis by excessive fibrotic reaction. This event sometimes makes difficult outpatient replacement of voice prosthesis and makes it necessary to use a lower diameter prosthesis (Fig. 4.8).

4.2.3   Granulation Tissue

About 5% of patients suffer from granulation tissue formation, often related to a concurrent infection. Dragicevic et al. suggest that blood on the tip of the brush during the cleaning of the prosthesis may be an indirect indicator of the presence of granulation tissue on the esophageal side of the TEP [1] or an indicator of the sealing of the esophageal flange in the thickness of the tracheoesophageal wall.

Fig. 4.7 Modification of
tracheostoma after surgery
for tracheal stenotic ring

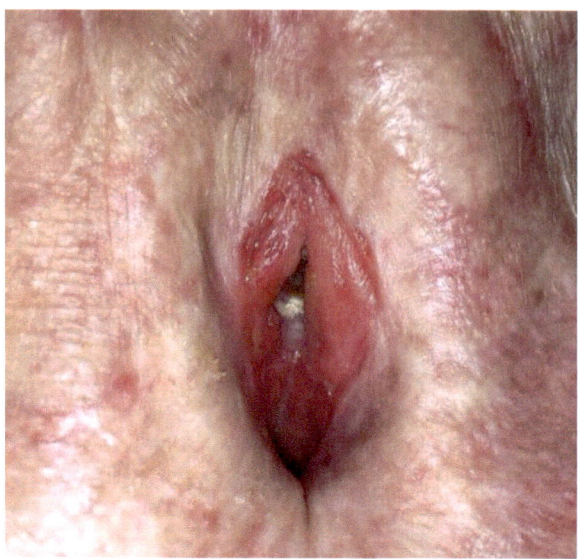

Fig. 4.8 Fibrotic stenosis
of tracheoesophageal
puncture: white fibrotic
ring (arrow)

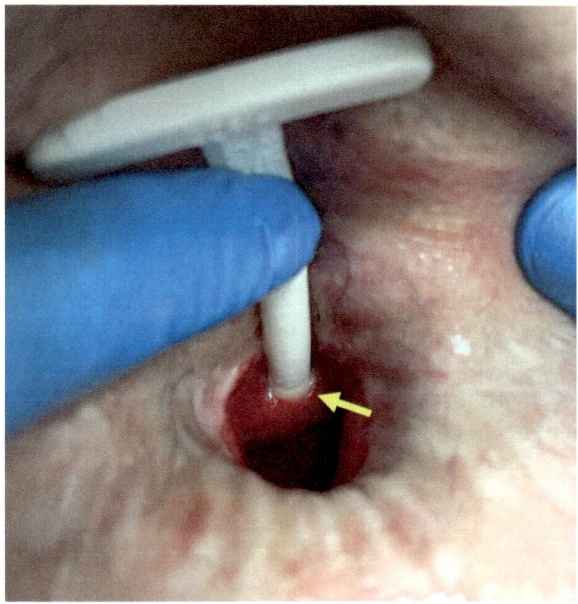

   If the granulation tissue is on the tracheal side, proper medical therapy or granulation exeresis is recommended [17]. The main consequence of granulation is the
dislocation of the voice prosthesis that can occur both on the tracheal side with
incarceration of the anterior flange (Fig. 4.9), and on the esophageal side with incarceration of the back flange in the thickness of the tracheoesophageal wall. In these

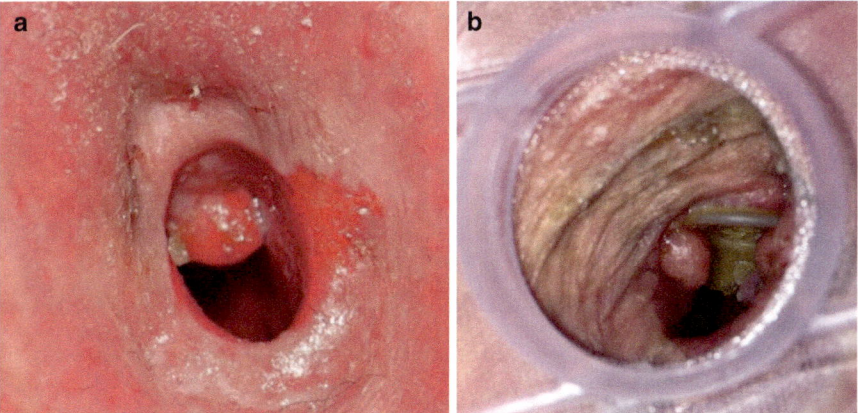

Fig. 4.9 Granulation tissue on tracheal side of tracheoesophageal puncture

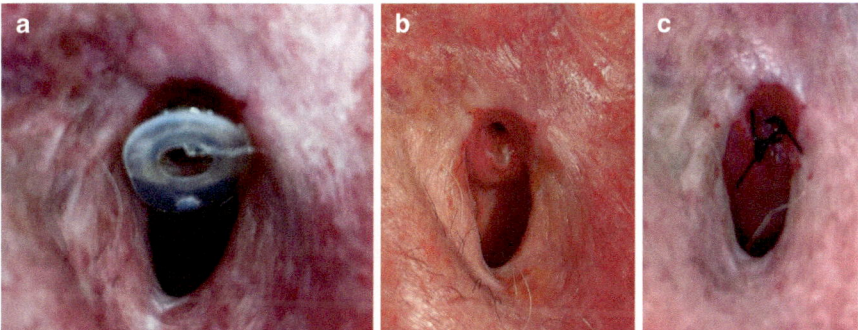

Fig. 4.10 Incarceration of esophageal flange with prosthesis extrusion (**a**), removal of prosthesis (**b**), and direct closure of tracheoesophageal puncture with suture (**c**)

cases, if possible, the VP is replaced by one of greater or equal length. However, sometimes, if the fistula is obliterated on one of the two sides, it is necessary to remove the prosthesis (Fig. 4.10) and perform a secondary TEP [18].

Rarely, the dislocation of the esophageal flange in the thickness of the tracheo-esophageal wall can lead to the onset of a pseudo-diverticulum, the so-called esophageal pouch, due to the detachment of the tracheal wall from the esophageal one [19, 20] (Fig. 4.11).

4.2.4   Peri-prosthetic Bleeding

Peri-prosthetic bleeding may occur during replacement procedures of voice prosthesis, especially if there are granulations. However, the bleeding usually terminates spontaneously at the end of the procedure.

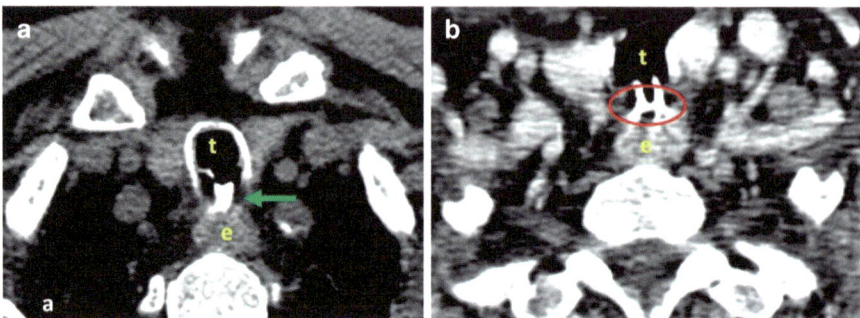

Fig. 4.11 Tracheal dislocation of voice prosthesis (green arrow) (**a**), esophageal pouch (red circle) (**b**) (*t* trachea, *e* esophagus)

Fig. 4.12 Peri-prosthetic hemorrhage in patient under anticoagulant therapy

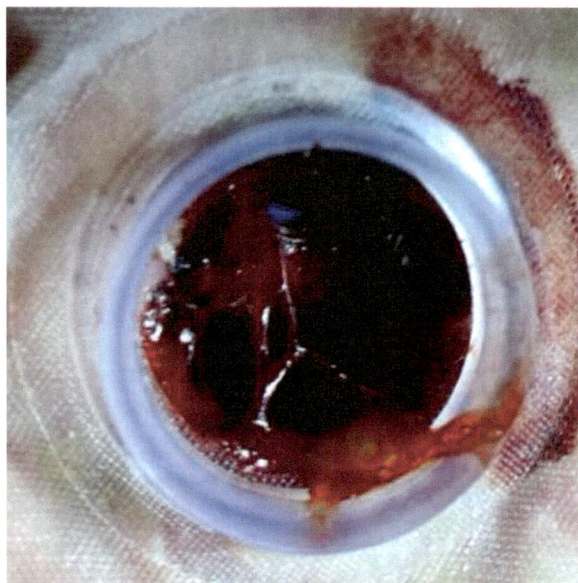

Occurrence of peri-prosthetic bleeding as a complication of secondary TEP in patients taking anticoagulants or antiplatelet drugs is less common but more serious (Fig. 4.12).

4.2.5   Aspiration or Ingestion of Voice Prosthesis

As previously written, a large TEP may cause—although rarely—the dislocation of the voice prosthesis resulting in its ingestion or aspiration [1].

The ingestion of the device is more frequent than the tracheal aspiration because the esophageal flange is thicker and stiffer than the tracheal one. In case of misplaced voice prosthesis, imaging, such as computed tomography (CT), is important to confirm its presence in the bowel.

Aspiration of voice prosthesis is less common (4–6% of cases) and represents an emergency to be treated promptly: the patient complains of coughing, breathlessness and may develop acute respiratory failure. In these cases, a chest X-ray or better chest CT should be performed to detect the voice prosthesis in the bronchus and then proceed to its removal by flexible or rigid bronchoscopy, forceps, and retrieval basket [21, 22]. Regarding imaging, all speech prostheses are radiopaque, especially those with a radiopaque ring; however, a chest X-ray often does not show the voice prosthesis, so the CT is more sensitive [2]. For anatomical reasons, the voice prosthesis is most frequently found in the right main bronchus since it has a larger diameter, and it is less angled than the left one.

Tong et al. defined the ingestion and inhalation of the VP as patient-related complications. In particular, they have imputed the ingestion of a VP as improper care of patients, e.g., over-vigorous cleaning with brush [2]. Inhalation of VP is instead more likely related to the patient in terms of manual and/or cognitive skills.

4.2.6   Too Low or Too High TEP

The position of the tracheoesophageal puncture is correct when it allows easy daily care by the patient as well as a simple and without trouble outpatient replacement of the VP [23]. Therefore, when creating the TEP, close attention should be paid to the TEP position relative to the tracheostoma. Indeed, a fistula too low compared to the level of tracheostoma makes cleaning it with a brush difficult or even impossible—with accidental risk of aspiration of the same brush—and requires retrograde replacement of the prosthesis (Fig. 4.13). The management of the fistula too high is equally difficult (Fig. 4.14). However, between the two events, managing the latter

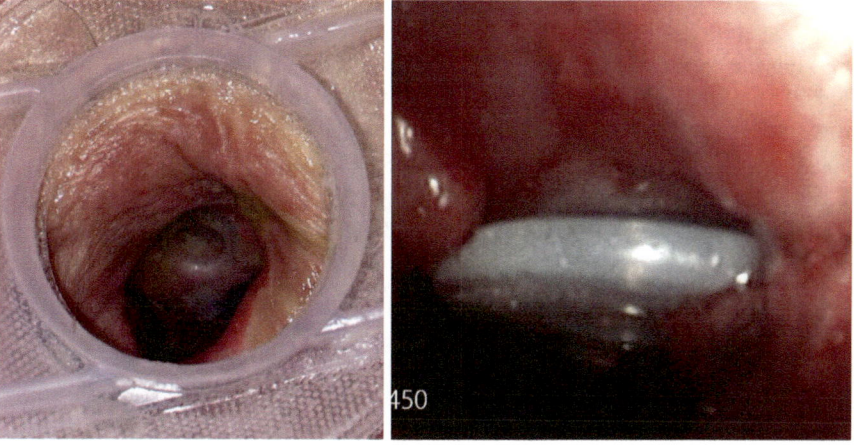

Fig. 4.13   Too low tracheoesophageal fistula

Fig. 4.14 Too high tracheoesophageal fistula

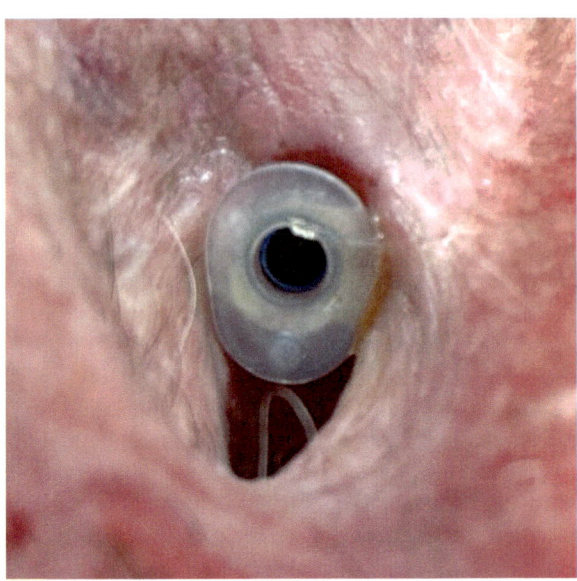

is easier than handling a too low fistula, without considering its optimal performance.

In these cases, the only solution is the closure of the TEP and later the creation of the TEP in the correct position according to tracheostoma features.

4.3   Complications Related to Voice Prosthesis

4.3.1   Incontinence of Voice Prosthesis (Trans-prosthetic Leakage)

Complications related to speech prosthesis inevitably lead to a leakage of fluid through the prosthesis, the so-called trans-prosthetic leakage. This occurrence is linked to normal and physiological "aging" and deterioration of the VP and therefore, according to some authors, it should not be considered a complication but the signal that the VP needs to be changed because it is no longer working properly, and it is no longer continent [3].

The causes of deterioration of the speech prosthesis are as follows:

– *Bacterial and/or fungal colonization of voice prosthesis*

The incontinence of the VP that results in leakage of fluid through the prosthesis is substantially due to its colonization by a biofilm of bacteria and fungi that deteriorate the device itself (Fig. 4.15) [24].

Bacterial and/or fungal colonization of voice prosthesis represents the main cause of its replacement in up to 80% of the cases [25]. It is an event that virtually

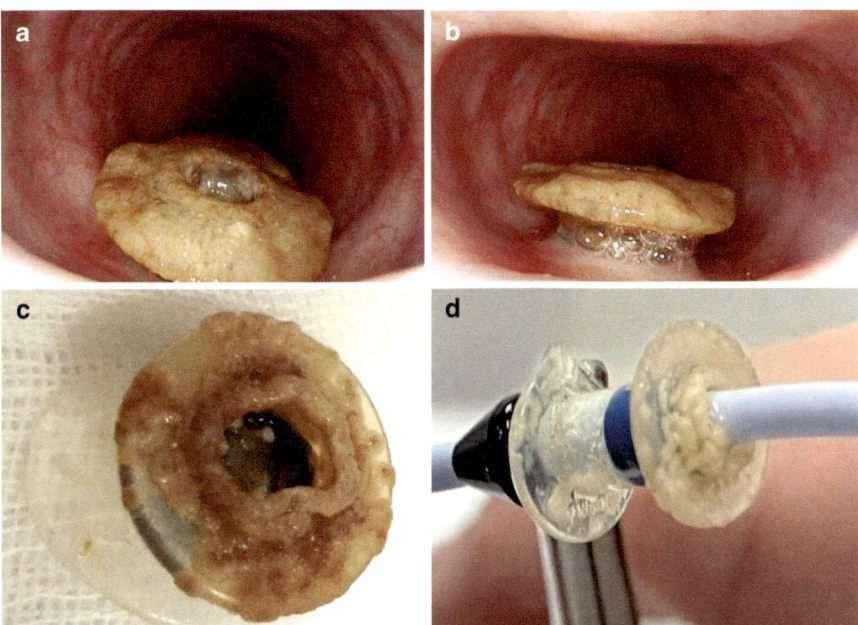

Fig. 4.15 Esophageal flange colonization

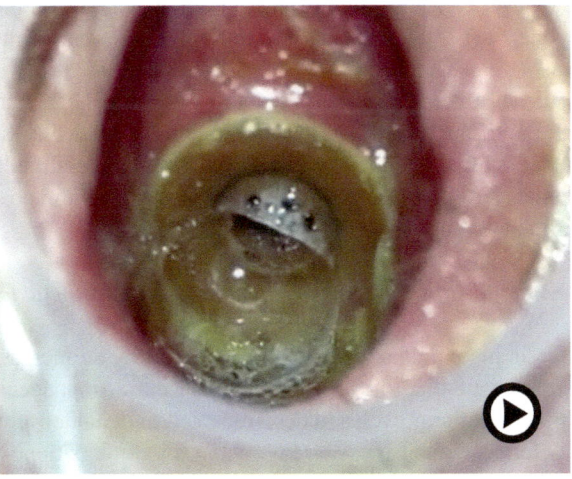

Fig. 4.16 Tracheal   flange   colonization   with   trans-prosthetic   leakage
(▶ https://doi.org/10.1007/000-bmt)

occurs in every patient and that can lead to malfunction of the prosthesis over time with peri- or trans-prosthetic leakage (Fig. 4.16) and therefore the need to replace the prosthesis itself. Several studies have reported that the esophageal flange of the VP is more frequently colonized by *Staphylococcus aureus*, among bacteria, and by *Candida albicans*, among fungi [26].

Fig. 4.17 Distortion of esophageal flange due to high intra-esophageal pressure

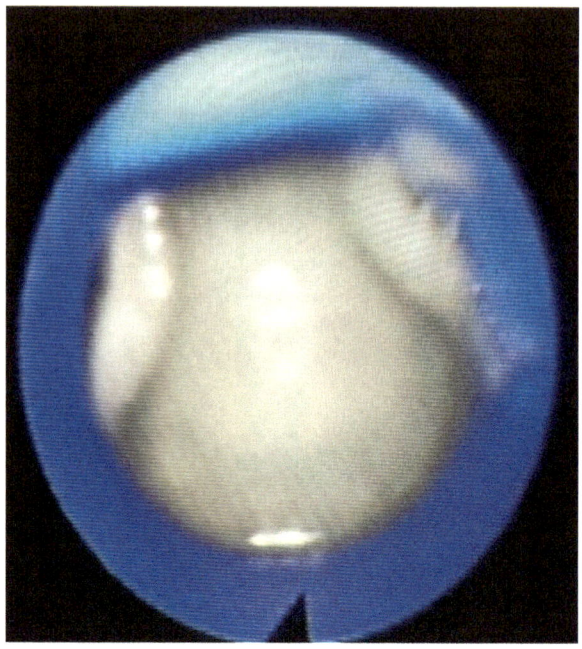

To prevent this occurrence, which would affect the average life of the VP (less than 2 months on average), topical antifungal drugs may be recommended, such as nystatin or fluconazole [27]. However, this strategy could promote the development of resistant yeast strains. A 2015 study showed that the fungal colonization of the speech prosthesis has a statistically significant role on the VP life span; however, the systematic use of antifungal solution does not improve statistically significantly the device life [28]. For this reason, in this case, the use of modified VP is recommended, since thanks to its features (silver oxide and/or titanium coating) [29] prevent local microbial colonization.

– *Reduced average life of the device due to early trans-prosthetic leakage*

Voice prosthesis incontinence is sometimes caused by an increased esophageal pressure. This rare issue due to cyclic increases in intra-esophageal pressure synchronous with the breathing cycles. These repeated and sudden pressure changes involve rapid deterioration of the VP (Fig. 4.17). In some patients, a decrease in intra-esophageal pressure occurs during each inhalation leading to the opening of the valve (about 22,000 cycles a day), with early deterioration of the speech prosthesis and consequent trans-valve leakage [1] (Figs. 4.18 and 4.19). Moreover, this increase in intra-esophageal pressure is found more commonly in patients undergoing secondary TEP in which the cricopharyngeal muscle myotomy has not been performed [15].

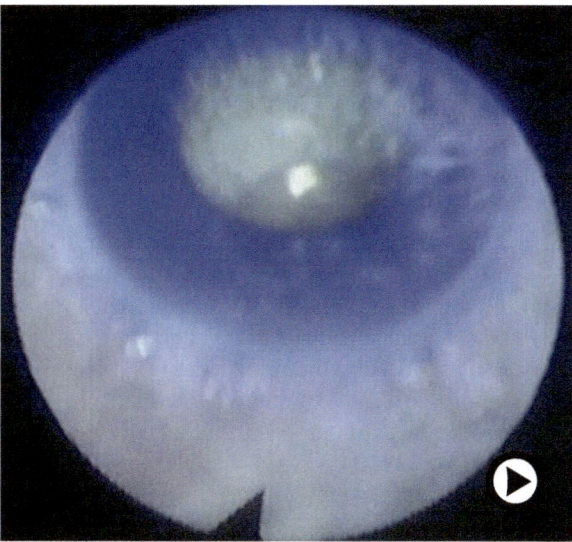

Fig. 4.18 Intra-esophageal pressure changes synchronous with breathing (tracheal view) (▶ https://doi.org/10.1007/000-bms)

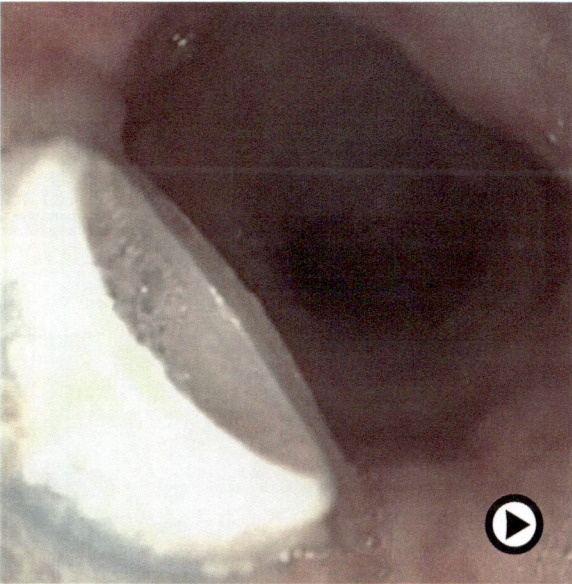

Fig. 4.19 Intra-esophageal pressure changes synchronous with breathing (esophageal view) (▶ https://doi.org/10.1007/000-bmv)

4.4   Complications Not Related to TEP or Voice Prosthesis

4.4.1   Pharyngeal Stricture/Stenosis/Spasm

Pharyngeal stricture occurs in about 30% of patients undergoing total laryngectomy and in about 50% of patients undergoing adjuvant RT [30–32]. In the first case, it is due to the failure of cricopharyngeal myotomy and/or neurotomy of the pharyngeal plexus during surgery resulting in pharyngeal hypertonicity (Fig. 4.20). RT, instead, provoke tissue fibrosis resulting in stiffness of the pharyngoesophageal lumen. In this situation, first, the patient complains of dysphagia (especially if the esophageal lumen has a diameter less than 12 mm) and later he complains also of difficult voice emission, feasible only with significant expiratory effort. The most effective therapy in the case of pharyngeal stenosis is the dilation of neopharynx: this procedure is usually performed in sedation and has a high success rate [33, 34].

4.4.2   Narrow Tracheostoma

The size and characteristics of tracheostoma play a primary role in ensuring a successful voice production through the VP as well as the simple and easy management of the TEP. Indeed, a narrow tracheostoma may correlate with dyspnea, difficulty in secretions aspiration, in the cleaning of the prosthesis and, above all, in its outpatient replacement (Fig. 4.21).

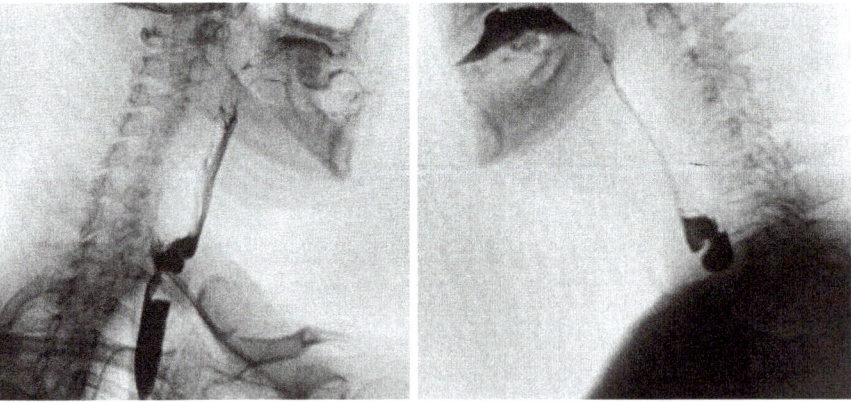

Fig. 4.20 Pharyngeal spasm due to cricopharyngeal hypertonicity (videofluorography)

Fig. 4.21 Consequences
of narrow stoma

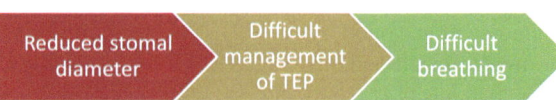

Reduced stomal diameter → Difficult management of TEP → Difficult breathing

Fig. 4.22 Decubitus lesion in narrowed stoma

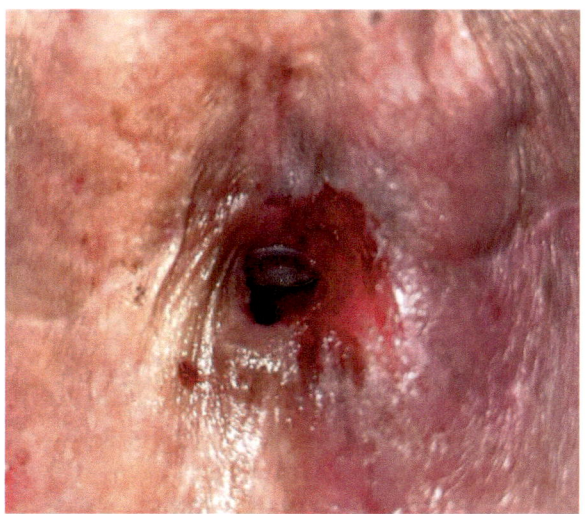

a   **b**

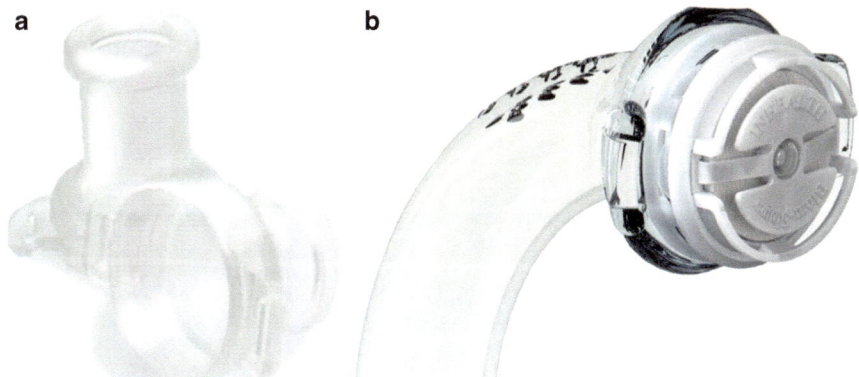

Fig. 4.23 Stoma button (**a**); silicon tube (**b**)

Sometimes, the excessive digital pressure on Heat and Moisture Exchanger (HME), due to phonatory effort, may cause peristomal skin decubitus lesions (Fig. 4.22).

In these situations, different strategies can be carried out according to the individual clinical case and the size of the tracheostoma. So, to prevent further narrowing of the tracheostoma, the patient can use the stoma button or, if stenosis also affects the tracheal lumen, he can use the silicone fenestrated tracheal tube (Fig. 4.23). The latter ensures the patency and size of trachea and tracheostoma, that being made of silicone, is more comfortable for the patient.

In more severe cases, a surgery to widen the tracheostoma should be performed. Over the years, different techniques have been proposed: "doughnut method," positioning a skin flap in the posterior wall of the upper trachea, "lateral flap technique" performing a double Z-plasty or a double V-Y plasty [35–37], "petal" technique

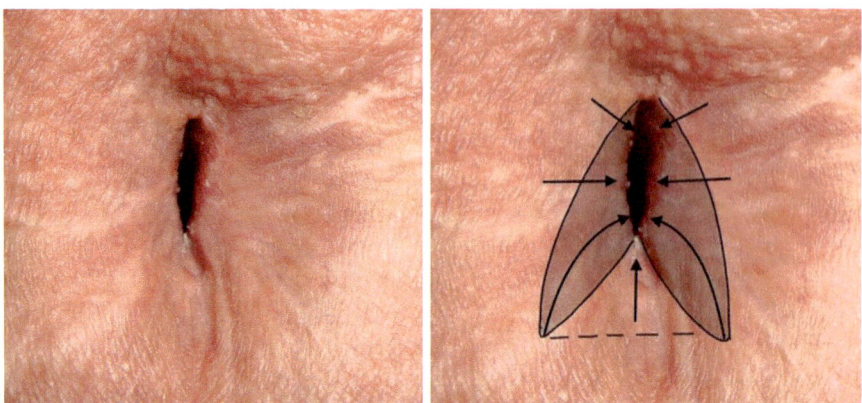

Fig. 4.24 Petal technique

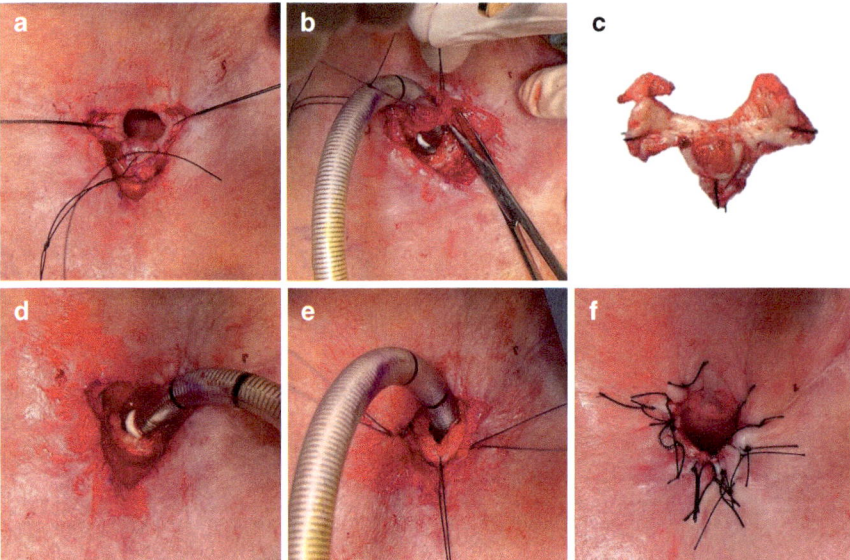

Fig. 4.25 Three-flap technique: (**a**) incision of three flaps of peristomal skin; (**b**) removal of the flaps including the stenotic tracheal ring; (**c**) three flaps removed specimen; (**d**) stoma before suture; (**e**) packaging of tracheostoma; (**f**) completed tracheostoma

[38], three-flap technique. These latter two are the most widely used techniques as they ensure better results. The "petal" technique consists in the removal of two petals of skin and subcutaneous oriented downwards together with the stenotic tracheal rings (2–3 rings). Then a vertical incision is made on the front wall of the trachea (encompassing 2 tracheal rings), and the dissected edges of the trachea are sutured with the apex of the triangle of skin removed (Fig. 4.24).

The three-flap technique consists in the removal of three flaps of peristomal skin together with the stenotic tracheal ring and in the subsequent packaging of the tracheostoma, thus obtaining a wider stoma (Figs. 4.25 and 4.26). In any case, after the

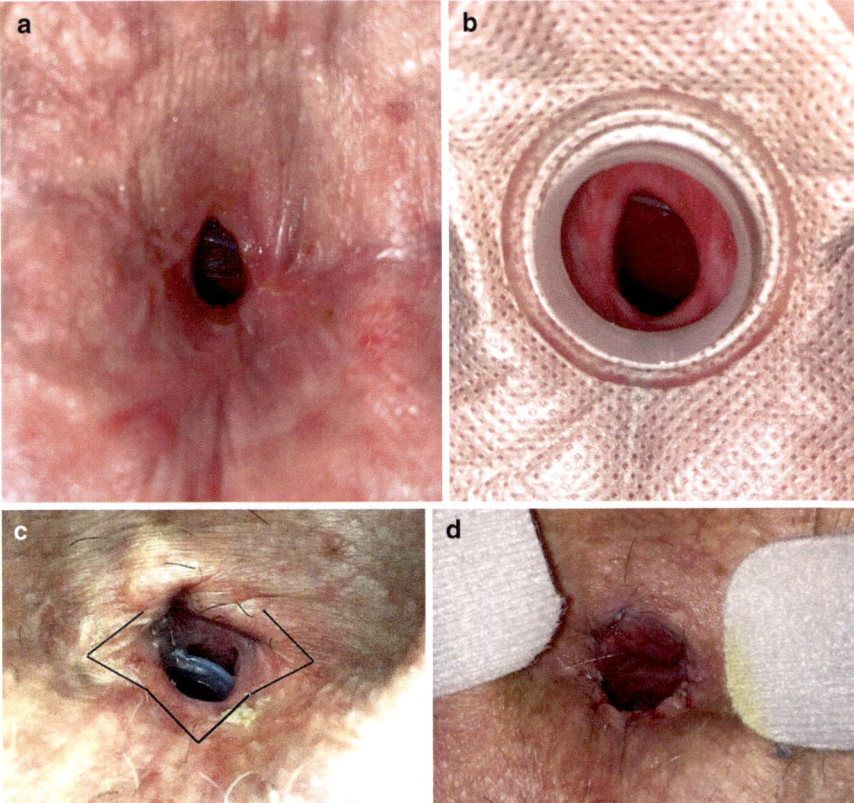

Fig. 4.26 Three-flap technique: case #1 before (**a**) and after (**b**) surgery; case #2 before (**c**) and after (**d**) surgery

enlargement surgery, the placement of the silicone tracheal tube is indicated until complete healing.

As described in the previous chapter, some precautions during the total laryngectomy should be followed to prevent this complication, thus avoiding the interruption of the cartilaginous rings [39], performing a meticulous suture of the skin to the trachea in order to cover the tracheal rings, and reducing the duration of the tracheal tube in post-operative [40]. Another prevention strategy was proposed by Suzuki et al. in 2010 [41]. The authors suggested preservation of the integrity of the posterior wall of the trachea and the oblique incision of the anterior wall of the trachea which is then sutured owered in order to achieve an "upside-down triangle" tracheostoma.

4.4.3 Deep Tracheostoma

Deep tracheostoma is defined as its placement in a depression limited by the protrusion of the two sternocleidomastoid muscles on the sides and by the manubrium of the sternum at the bottom (Fig. 4.27).

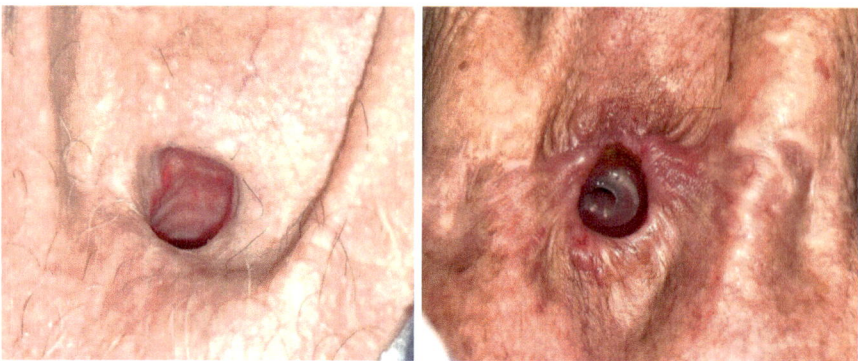

Fig. 4.27 Deep tracheostoma

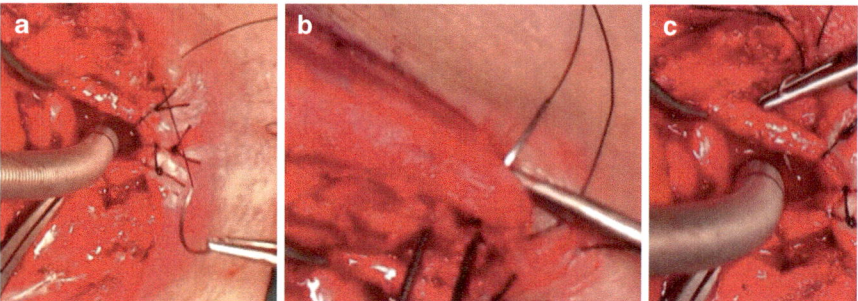

Fig. 4.28 Creation of the tracheostoma: stitch including skin (**a**), sternocleidomastoid muscle (**b**), and tracheal ring (**c**)

For this reason, the correct positioning of the peristomal adhesive patch and of the HME and therefore, the adequate respiratory and phonatory rehabilitation turn out to be difficult. A 2011 study showed that the use of the patch is more frequent in patients with flat tracheostoma, instead it is little used by patients with tilted backward and deep tracheostoma [42].

To prevent this eventuality, Santoro et al. suggest the section of the sternal head of the sternocleidomastoid (SCM) muscles during total laryngectomy surgery [43]. Otherwise, as described in the previous chapter, the sternal head of the sternocleidomastoid muscles can be sutured and made integral to the lateral wall of the trachea in order to ensure the flattening and the stability over time of the tracheostoma (Fig. 4.28).

In this regard, a 2011 study analyzed the role that different parameters could play on morphology and geometry of tracheostoma: horizontal and vertical diameter of the tracheostoma, neck circumference at tracheostoma level, distance between sternocleidomastoid muscles, distance between upper edge of tracheostoma and hyoid bone, distance between the lower edge of the tracheostoma and the jugulum, distance between lateral edges of the tracheostoma and SCM muscles, and upper and lower edge depth of the tracheostoma. This multicentric analysis showed that

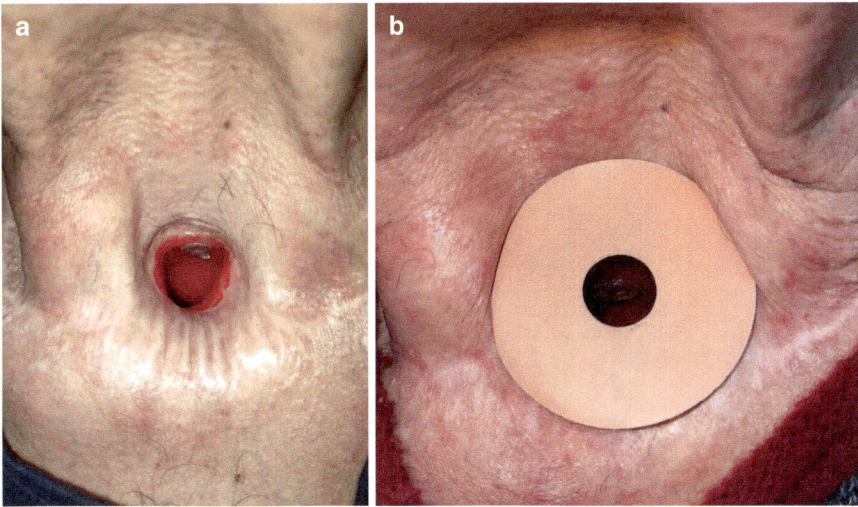

Fig. 4.29 Deep tracheostoma (**a**) and self-adhesive silicon pad to level out the tracheostoma (**b**)

neither the section of the sternal head of SCM muscle nor the number of tracheal rings removed affects the development or not of a deep tracheostoma [44]. However, if the patient presents a deep tracheostoma and none of the measures outlined above has been previously carried out, a revision surgery can be performed, e.g., the myotomy of sternal head of sternocleidomastoid muscle, under local anesthesia [43], or tracheal suspension. On the other hand, the non-surgical strategy is the self-adhesive silicon pad which, placed below the peristomal patch, allows to level out the tracheostoma (Fig. 4.29).

4.5 Troubles in Voice Emission

4.5.1 Excessive Length of Voice Prosthesis

Normally, the tracheal and esophageal flanges of the VP should rest on the back wall of the trachea and on the anterior wall of the esophagus, respectively. In the case of too long VP, looking through the tracheostoma, you will see not only the tracheal flange but also part of the shaft of the VP. This condition often occurs due to reduction of post-surgical edema, after the surgery for the creation of the TEP and placement of the speech prosthesis. Another cause is the tissue atrophy resulting in thinning of the TEP tract (Fig. 4.30), e.g., due to radiation therapy [7].

The presence of a too long speech prostheses is related to a high risk of periprosthetic leakage (Fig. 4.31).

Moreover, in these situations, during the digital occlusion of the stoma, the prosthesis can be pushed against the posterior esophageal wall resulting in obstruction of the trans-prosthetic airflow. This repeated trauma can lead to the development of

Fig. 4.30 Thinning of
tracheoesophageal tract

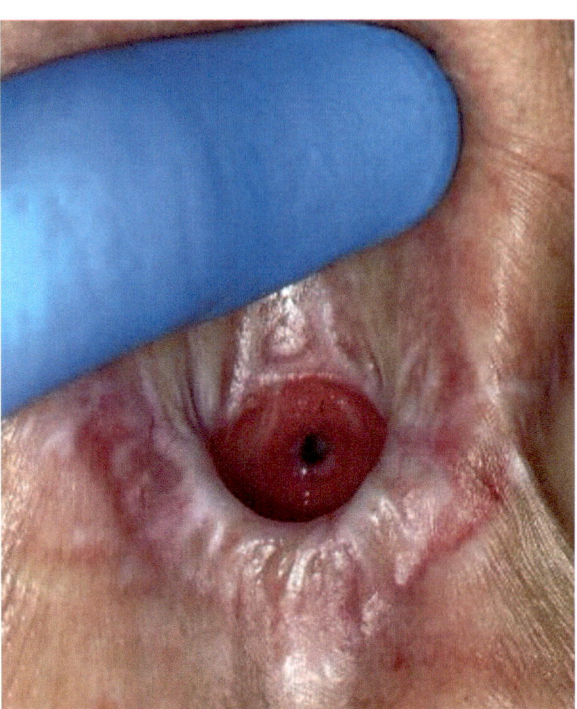

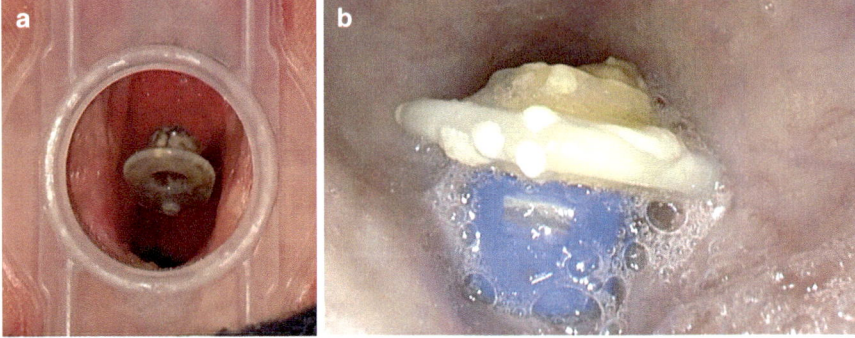

Fig. 4.31 Too long voice prosthesis: tracheal view (**a**) and esophageal view (**b**)

pressure sores up to necrosis of the posterior esophageal wall. The replacement of a
shorter voice prosthesis allows a solution to the problem [25] (Fig. 4.32).

4.5.2 Short Voice Prosthesis

In some cases, during the outpatient examination, the opposite to the previous condition can be found, namely a too short voice prosthesis or, more correctly, a thickening of the tracheoesophageal wall that has partially incorporated the prosthesis
itself (Figs. 4.33 and 4.34).

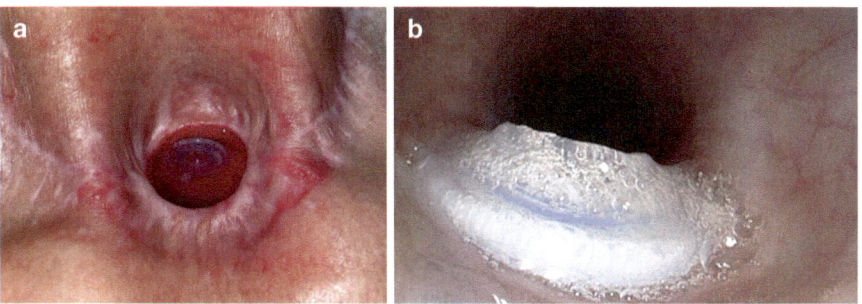

Fig. 4.32 Correct fitting of voice prosthesis: tracheal view (**a**) and esophageal view (**b**)

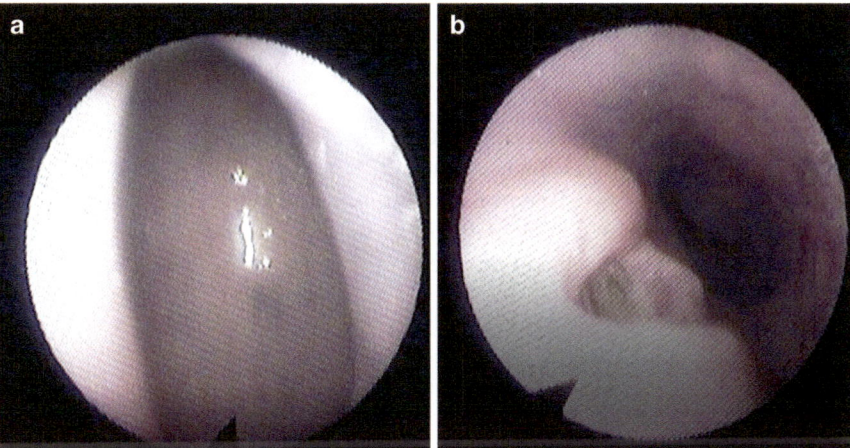

Fig. 4.33 Short voice prosthesis with its partially incorporation in the tracheoesophageal wall: trans-prosthetic view (**a**) and esophageal view (**b**)

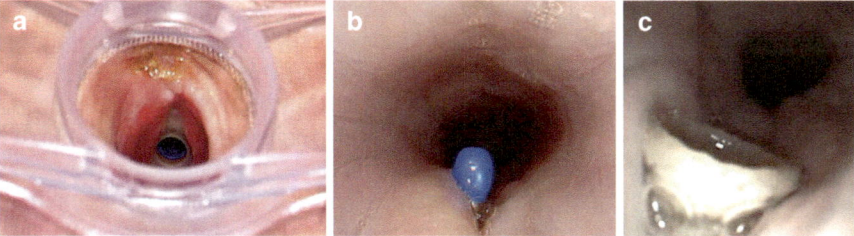

Fig. 4.34 Short voice prosthesis: tracheal flange covered by tracheal mucosa (**a**), esophageal flange completely covered by esophageal mucosa

Hypertrophy of the TEP tract often results from infection or chronic trauma due to excessive pressure on the prosthesis during phonation. In these cases, both the tracheal and the esophageal flanges of the VP are covered by mucosa making its replacement also difficult. Moreover, this condition correlates to progressive

Fig. 4.35 Videofluorography
showing pharyngeal
hypertonicity

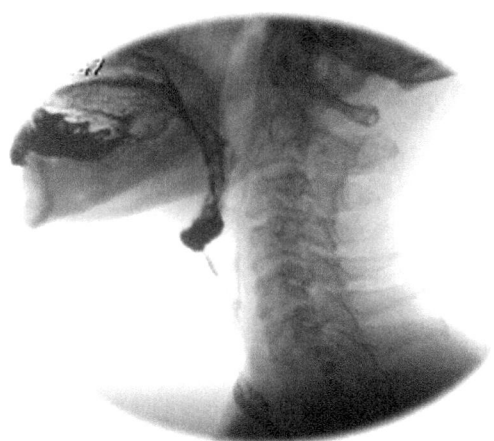

dislocation up to ingestion of the prosthesis as well as to the risk of detachment of the tracheal wall from the esophageal one [19].

In these situations, two aspects need to be addressed: replacing a longer voice prosthesis and solving the problem that led to the thickening of the TEP tract, e.g., with vocal rest, antibiotic, and/or oral steroidal therapy.

4.5.3   Pharyngeal Hypertonicity

Some patients may report difficult phonation, possible only with significant expiratory effort. In some cases, patients may also complain of dysphagia. This condition is often due to hypertonicity of the pharyngeal-esophageal segment (PES) and may manifest immediately after the placement of the device or later. Diagnosis can be made through several instrumental examinations such as electromyography (EMG), endoscopy, videofluorography, and manometry [45]. In particular, esophageal videofluorography shows a stricture (due to hypertonia) at PES level with reduced or, in some cases almost completely absent, passage of the bolus of barium sulfate (Fig. 4.35).

Once the location of the PES stricture or spasm has been radiologically identified, lidocaine infiltrations are transcutaneously performed. After about 5 min, the vocal emission by voice prosthesis is evaluated: if the patient can speak effortlessly, it means that the problem has been correctly identified and that the resolution therapy can be carried out. In this case, therapy is represented by infiltrations of botulinum toxin A (BTA) in order to relax the cricopharyngeal muscle and the upper esophageal sphincter (UES) (Fig. 4.36).

BTA infiltrations are usually performed transcutaneously, preferably under EMG control. Indeed, the electromyographic control of the procedure guarantees to infiltrate the muscle rather than the surrounding fibrous tissue. In 2009, Krause et al. performed endoscopic infiltrations under general anesthesia, proving that this approach allows a direct visual control of the inoculum site of the drug with

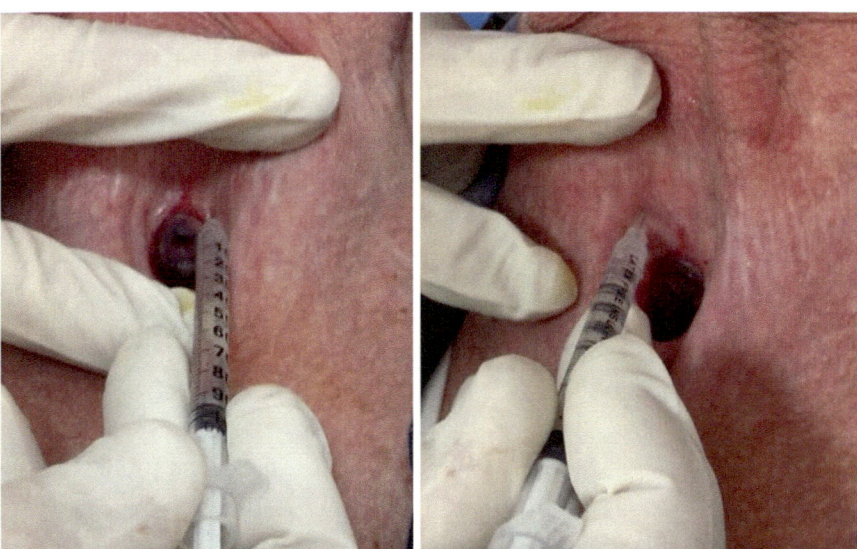

Fig. 4.36 Transcutaneously infiltration of botulinum toxin A

minimal risk of complications [46]. The effect of BTA begins about 2–3 days after infiltration and lasts about 3–6 months, then the procedure should be repeated. Therefore, despite the advantages presented by Krause et al. its approach is not advisable since it means that the patient must undergo general anesthesia 2–4 times a year. However, studies have shown a progressive reduction in the number of required infiltrations over the years probably due to a progressive hypotonia of the pharyngeal muscles [47]. This treatment also seems to increase the life of the VP since it reduces the effort during phonation [46].

As described in the previous chapter, performing unilateral myotomy of the cricopharyngeal muscle [48] and/or unilateral pharyngeal plexus neurectomy [49] during total laryngectomy surgery is advisable to avoid hypertonia of PES, both in case of primary and secondary TEP.

4.5.4 Pharyngoesophageal Hypotonia

Hypotonia of pharyngoesophageal segment involves the production of a weak and whispered voice. Sometimes the cause is unclear, other times is due to a surgical error during total laryngectomy, namely the myotomy of both cricopharyngeal muscles. Also on this occasion, videofluorography enables to achieve a diagnosis of certainty: X-ray images show PES dilation with barium accumulation (Fig. 4.37). In these cases, it is important to reduce the size of the lumen of the PES by exerting external pressure with an elastic band to wrap the neck or surgically using the sternocleidomastoid muscles as an "internal pressure band" [50]. Moreover, the use of a higher resistance voice prosthesis can improve the phonation [51].

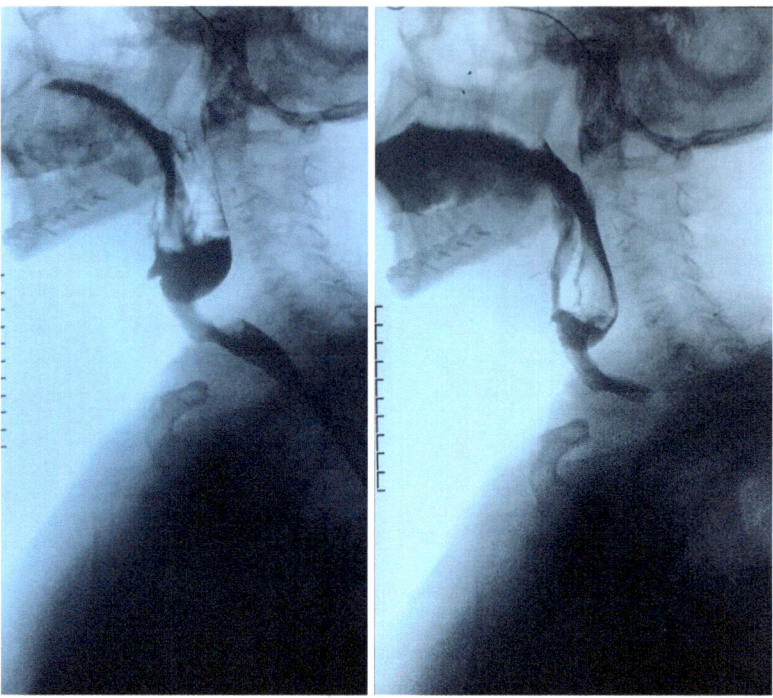

Fig. 4.37 Videofluorography showing pharyngeal hypotonia

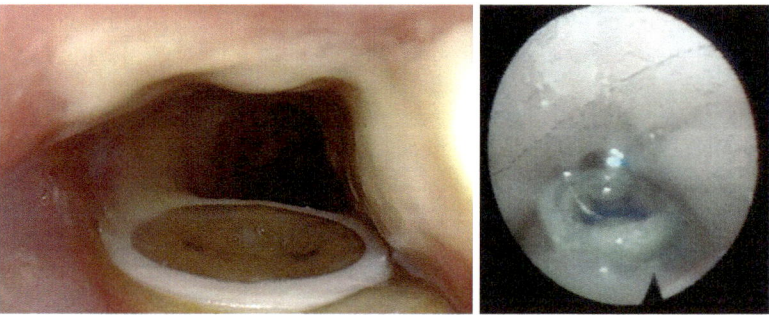

Fig. 4.38 Pressure sores of the posterior esophageal wall

4.5.5 Pressure Sores or Necrosis of the Posterior Esophageal Wall

As mentioned above, a voice prosthesis too long, excessive digital pressure on the HME during phonation and/or the persistent pressure exerted by the endotracheal tube on the VP can cause pressure sores up to necrosis of the posterior esophageal wall (Fig. 4.38).

Declaration by Authors Figures are original and free from copyright issues.

References

1. Dragicevic DM, Jovic RM, Kljajic VL, Vlaski LM, Savovic SN, Lemajic-Komazec SN. Complications following secondary voice prosthesis insertion and impact of previous irradiation on their appearance. Niger J Clin Pract. 2021;24(4):470–5. https://doi.org/10.4103/njcp.njcp_549_19.
2. Tong JY, Pasick LJ, Benito DA, Sataloff RT. Complications associated with tracheoesophageal voice prostheses from 2010 to 2020: a MAUDE study. Am J Otolaryngol. 2020;41(6):102652. https://doi.org/10.1016/j.amjoto.2020.102652. Epub 2020 Jul 17.
3. Scherl C, Kauffels J, Schützenberger A, Döllinger M, Bohr C, Dürr S, Fietkau R, Haderlein M, Koch M, Traxdorf M, Mantsopoulos K, Müller S, Iro H. Secondary tracheoesophageal puncture after laryngectomy increases complications with shunt and voice prosthesis. Laryngoscope. 2020;130(12):E865–73. https://doi.org/10.1002/lary.28517. Epub 2020 Feb 6.
4. Petersen JF, Lansaat L, Timmermans AJ, van der Noort V, Hilgers FJM, van den Brekel MWM. Postlaryngectomy prosthetic voice rehabilitation outcomes in a consecutive cohort of 232 patients over a 13-year period. Head Neck. 2019;41(3):623–31. https://doi.org/10.1002/hed.25364. Epub 2019 Jan 7. PMID: 30614644; PMCID: PMC6590326.
5. Kress P, Schäfer P, Schwerdtfeger FP. Die custom-fit-Stimmprothese. Zur Therapie der periprothetischen Leckage bei Stimmprothesenträgern [the custom-fit voice prosthesis, for treatment of periprosthetic leakage after tracheoesophageal voice restoration]. Laryngorhinootologie. 2006;85(7):496–500. https://doi.org/10.1055/s-2006-925081. Epub 2006 Feb 21.
6. Lundy DS, Landera MA, Bremekamp J, Weed D. Longitudinal tracheoesophageal puncture size stability. Otolaryngol Head Neck Surg. 2012;147(5):885–8. https://doi.org/10.1177/0194599812449293. Epub 2012 May 22.
7. Choussy O, Hibon R, Bon Mardion N, Dehesdin D. Management of voice prosthesis leakage with Blom-Singer large esophage and tracheal flange voice prostheses. Eur Ann Otorhinolaryngol Head Neck Dis. 2013;130(2):49–53. https://doi.org/10.1016/j.anorl.2012.03.008. Epub 2012 Nov 24.
8. Rodríguez-Lorenzana P, Mayo-Yáñez M, Chiesa-Estomba CM, Vaira LA, Lechien JR, Maniaci A, Cabo-Varela I. Cost-effectiveness study of double-flange voice prostheses in the treatment of periprosthetic leakage in laryngectomized patients. J Pers Med. 2023;13(7):1064. https://doi.org/10.3390/jpm13071064.
9. Jacobs K, Delaere PR, Vander Poorten VL. Submucosal purse-string suture as a treatment of leakage around the indwelling voice prosthesis. Head Neck. 2008;30(4):485–91. https://doi.org/10.1002/hed.20732.
10. Bozec A, Poissonnet G, Chamorey E, Demard F, Santini J, Peyrade F, Ortholan C, Benezery K, Thariat J, Sudaka A, Anselme K, Adrey B, Giacchero P, Dassonville O. Results of vocal rehabilitation using tracheoesophageal voice prosthesis after total laryngectomy and their predictive factors. Eur Arch Otorrinolaringol. 2010;267(5):751–8. https://doi.org/10.1007/s00405-009-1138-x. Epub 2009 Nov 5.
11. Parrilla C, Almadori A, Longobardi Y, Lattanzi W, Salgarello M, Almadori G. Regenerative strategy for persistent periprosthetic leakage around tracheoesophageal puncture: is it an effective long-term solution? Cell. 2021;10(7):1695. https://doi.org/10.3390/cells10071695.
12. Saeedi A, Strum DP, Mir G, Chow MS, Bhatt N, Jacobson AS. Management of enlarging tracheoesophageal fistula with voice prosthesis in laryngectomized patients. Laryngoscope. 2023;134:198. https://doi.org/10.1002/lary.30857. Epub ahead of print.
13. Parrilla C, Longobardi Y, Galli J, Rigante M, Paludetti G, Bussu F, Scarano E. Periprosthetic leakage in tracheoesophageal prosthesis: proposal of a standardized therapeutic algorithm. Otolaryngol Head Neck Surg. 2021;165(3):446–54. https://doi.org/10.1177/0194599820983343. Epub 2021 Jan 5.
14. Zhang T, Maclean J, Szczesniak M, Bertrand PP, Quon H, Tsang RK, Wu PI, Graham P, Cook IJ. Esophageal dysmotility in patients following total laryngectomy. Otolaryngol Head Neck Surg. 2018;158(2):323–30. https://doi.org/10.1177/0194599817736507. Epub 2017 Dec 12.

15. Danic Hadzibegovic A, Kozmar A, Hadzibegovic I, Prgomet D, Danic D. Influence of proton pump inhibitor therapy on occurrence of voice prosthesis complications. Eur Arch Otorrinolaringol. 2020;277(4):1177–84. https://doi.org/10.1007/s00405-020-05784-4. Epub 2020 Jan 17.

16. Hiltmann O, Buntrock M, Hagen R. Mechanischer Ileus durch Provox-Stimmprothese—Beschreibung einer "iatrogenen" enteralen Komplikation nach Stimmprothesenwechsel [Mechanical ileus caused by a Provox voice prosthesis—an "iatrogenic" enteral complication in voice prosthesis rehabilitation of laryngectomees]. Laryngorhinootologie. 2002;81(12):890–3. https://doi.org/10.1055/s-2002-36106.

17. Neumann A, Schultz-Coulon HJ. Management von Komplikationen nach prothetischer Stimmrehabilitation. [Management of complications after prosthetic voice rehabilitation]. HNO. 2000;48(7):508–16. https://doi.org/10.1007/s001060050607.

18. Yavuz H, Vural O. Tracheoesophageal puncture closure with annular mucosal flap. Head Neck. 2021;43(6):1705–10. https://doi.org/10.1002/hed.26631. Epub 2021 Feb 5.

19. Hoffman HT, Baker SR. Tracheostoma diverticulum following tracheoesophageal puncture. Arch Otolaryngol Head Neck Surg. 1990;116(9):1074–6. https://doi.org/10.1001/archotol.1990.01870090090015.

20. Saraniti C, Greco G, Verro B, Chianetta E, Lo-Casto A. Zenker's diverticulum in Forestier disease: chance or causality? Iran J Otorhinolaryngol. 2022;34(121):107–12. https://doi.org/10.22038/IJORL.2021.60053.3068.

21. Abia-Trujillo D, Tatari MM, Venegas-Borsellino CP, Hoffman RJ, Fox HT, Fernandez-Bussy I, Guru PK. Misplaced tracheoesophageal voice prosthesis: a case of foreign body aspiration. Am J Emerg Med. 2021;41:266.e1–2. https://doi.org/10.1016/j.ajem.2020.08.060. Epub 2020 Aug 28.

22. Conte SC, De Nardi E, Conte F, Nardini S. Aspiration of tracheoesophageal prosthesis in a laryngectomized patient. Multidiscip Respir Med. 2012;7(1):25. https://doi.org/10.1186/2049-6958-7-25.

23. Pighi GP, Barbieri F, Adami R, Fiorino F. Secondary tracheoesophageal puncture: blind technique with a rigid hysterometer. Laryngoscope. 2009;119(7):1431–4. https://doi.org/10.1002/lary.20518.

24. Apert V, Carsuzaa F, Tonnerre D, Leclerc J, Lebreton JP, Delagranda A, Dufour X. Speech restoration with tracheoesophageal prosthesis after total laryngectomy: an observational study of vocal results, complications and quality of life. Eur Ann Otorhinolaryngol Head Neck Dis. 2022;139(2):73–6. https://doi.org/10.1016/j.anorl.2021.05.008. Epub 2021 Jun 14.

25. Parrilla C, Longobardi Y, Paludetti G, Marenda ME, D'Alatri L, Bussu F, Scarano E, Galli J. A 1-year time frame for voice prosthesis management. What should the physician expect? Is it an overrated job? Acta Otorhinolaryngol Ital. 2020;40(4):270–6. https://doi.org/10.14639/0392-100X-N0587.

26. Rodrigues L, Banat IM, Teixeira J, Oliveira R. Strategies for the prevention of microbial biofilm formation on silicone rubber voice prostheses. J Biomed Mater Res B Appl Biomater. 2007;81(2):358–70. https://doi.org/10.1002/jbm.b.30673.

27. Pentland DR, Stevens S, Williams L, Baker M, McCall C, Makarovaite V, Balfour A, Mühlschlegel FA, Gourlay CW. Precision antifungal treatment significantly extends voice prosthesis lifespan in patients following total laryngectomy. Front Microbiol. 2020;11:975. https://doi.org/10.3389/fmicb.2020.00975.

28. Yenigun A, Eren SB, Ozkul MH, Tugrul S, Meric A. Factors influencing the longevity and replacement frequency of Provox voice prostheses. Singap Med J. 2015;56(11):632–6. https://doi.org/10.11622/smedj.2015173.

29. Talpaert MJ, Balfour A, Stevens S, Baker M, Muhlschlegel FA, Gourlay CW. Candida biofilm formation on voice prostheses. J Med Microbiol. 2015;64(Pt 3):199–208. https://doi.org/10.1099/jmm.0.078717-0. Epub 2014 Aug 8.

30. Vu KN, Day TA, Gillespie MB, Martin-Harris B, Sinha D, Stuart RK, Sharma AK. Proximal esophageal stenosis in head and neck cancer patients after total laryngectomy and radiation. ORL J Otorhinolaryngol Relat Spec. 2008;70(4):229–35. https://doi.org/10.1159/000130870. Epub 2008 May 9.

31. Kraaijenga SA, Oskam IM, van der Molen L, Hamming-Vrieze O, Hilgers FJ, van den Brekel MW. Evaluation of long term (10-years+) dysphagia and trismus in patients treated with concurrent chemo-radiotherapy for advanced head and neck cancer. Oral Oncol. 2015;51(8):787–94. https://doi.org/10.1016/j.oraloncology.2015.05.003. Epub 2015 May 28.

32. Massaro N, Verro B, Greco G, Chianetta E, D'Ecclesia A, Saraniti C. Quality of life with voice prosthesis after total laryngectomy. Iran J Otorhinolaryngol. 2021;33(118):301–9. https://doi.org/10.22038/ijorl.2021.53724.2832.

33. Petersen JF, Pézier TF, van Dieren JM, van der Noort V, van Putten T, Bril SI, Janssen L, Dirven R, van den Brekel MWM, de Bree R. Dilation after laryngectomy: incidence, risk factors and complications. Oral Oncol. 2019;91:107–12. https://doi.org/10.1016/j.oraloncology.2019.02.025. Epub 2019 Mar 6.

34. Piotet E, Escher A, Monnier P. Esophageal and pharyngeal strictures: report on 1862 endoscopic dilatations using the Savary-Gilliard technique. Eur Arch Otorrinolaringol. 2008;265(3):357–64. https://doi.org/10.1007/s00405-007-0456-0. Epub 2007 Sep 26.

35. Verschuur HP, Gregor RT, Hilgers FJ, Balm AJ. The tracheostoma in relation to prosthetic voice rehabilitation. Laryngoscope. 1996;106(1 Pt 1):111–5. https://doi.org/10.1097/00005537-199601000-00022.

36. Wax MK, Touma BJ, Ramadan HH. Tracheostomal stenosis revision with simultaneous tracheoesophageal puncture. Laryngoscope. 1998;108(10):1509–13. https://doi.org/10.1097/00005537-199810000-00015.

37. Panje WR, Kitt VV. Tracheal stoma reconstruction. Arch Otolaryngol. 1985;111(3):190–2. https://doi.org/10.1001/archotol.1985.00800050084013.

38. Lucioni M, Rizzotto G, Pazzaia T, Serafini I. Plastic tracheostomal-widening procedure: the "petal" technique. Acta Otorhinolaryngol Ital. 2003;23(4):291–6.

39. Lorenz KJ, Maier H. Pulmonale Rehabilitation nach totaler Laryngektomie durch die Verwendung von HME (Heat Moisture Exchanger) [Pulmonary rehabilitation after total laryngectomy using a heat and moisture exchanger (HME)]. Laryngorhinootologie. 2009;88(8):513–22. https://doi.org/10.1055/s-0029-1225619. Epub 2009 Jul 30.

40. Vlantis AC, Marres HA, van den Hoogen FJ. A surgical technique to prevent tracheostomal stenosis after laryngectomy. Laryngoscope. 1998;108(1 Pt 1):134–7. https://doi.org/10.1097/00005537-199801000-00026.

41. Suzuki M, Tsunoda A, Shirakura S, Sumi T, Nishijima W, Kishimoto S. A novel permanent tracheostomy technique for prevention of stomal stenosis (triangular tracheostomy). Auris Nasus Larynx. 2010;37(4):465–8. https://doi.org/10.1016/j.anl.2009.11.007. Epub 2009 Dec 29.

42. van der Houwen EB, van Kalkeren TA, Post WJ, Hilgers FJ, van der Laan BF, Verkerke GJ. Does the patch fit the stoma? A study on peristoma geometry and patch use in laryngectomized patients. Clin Otolaryngol. 2011;36(3):235–41. https://doi.org/10.1111/j.1749-4486.2011.02307.x.

43. Santoro GP, Luparello P, Lazio MS, Comini LV, Martelli F, Cannavicci A. Myotomy of sternocleidomastoid muscle as a secondary procedure in laryngectomized patients. Head Neck. 2019;41(10):3743–6. https://doi.org/10.1002/hed.25852. Epub 2019 Jul 26.

44. van Kalkeren TA, van der Houwen EB, Duits MA, Hilgers FJ, Hebe A, Mostafa BE, Lawson G, Martinez Z, Woisard V, Marioni G, Ruske D, Schultz P, Post WJ, Verkerke BJ, van der Laan BF. Worldwide, multicenter study of peristomal geometry and morphology in laryngectomees and its clinical effects. Head Neck. 2011;33(8):1184–90. https://doi.org/10.1002/hed.21595. Epub 2011 Mar 29.

45. Chone CT, Seixas VO, Andreollo NA, Quagliato E, Barcelos IH, Spina AL, Crespo AN. Computerized manometry use to evaluate spasm in pharyngoesophageal segment in patients with poor tracheoesophageal speech before and after treatment with botulinum toxin. Braz J Otorhinolaryngol. 2009;75(2):182–7. https://doi.org/10.1016/s1808-8694(15)30776-x.

46. Krause E, Hempel JM, Gürkov R. Botulinum toxin a prolongs functional durability of voice prostheses in laryngectomees with pharyngoesophageal spasm. Am J Otolaryngol. 2009;30(6):371–5. https://doi.org/10.1016/j.amjoto.2008.07.008. Epub 2009 Mar 9.

47. Ramachandran K, Arunachalam PS, Hurren A, Marsh RL, Samuel PR. Botulinum toxin injection for failed tracheo-oesophageal voice in laryngectomees: the Sunderland experience. J Laryngol Otol. 2003;117(7):544–8. https://doi.org/10.1258/002221503322112978.
48. Singer MI, Blom ED. Selective myotomy for voice restoration after total laryngectomy. Arch Otolaryngol. 1981;107(11):670–3. https://doi.org/10.1001/archotol.1981.00790470018005.
49. Singer MI, Blom ED, Hamaker RC. Pharyngeal plexus neurectomy for alaryngeal speech rehabilitation. Laryngoscope. 1986;96(1):50–4. https://doi.org/10.1288/00005537-198601000-00008.
50. Kapila M, Deore N, Palav RS, Kazi RA, Shah RP, Jagade MV. A brief review of voice restoration following total laryngectomy. Indian J Cancer. 2011;48(1):99–104. https://doi.org/10.4103/0019-509X.75841.
51. van Weissenbruch R, Kunnen M, Albers FW, van Cauwenberge PB, Sulter AM. Cineradiography of the pharyngoesophageal segment in postlaryngectomy patients. Ann Otol Rhinol Laryngol. 2000;109(3):311–9. https://doi.org/10.1177/000348940010900314.

In-Office Replacement of Voice Prosthesis

5.1   Introduction

There are two types of voice prosthesis (VP): indwelling and non-indwelling. The last of which rarely used are advantageous since they can be replaced directly by the patient without the need of the specialist but have a shorter life span than indwelling VP. Today, indwelling prostheses are predominantly used and are replaced on an outpatient basis by the specialist.

Like any device, the voice prosthesis has an average life that ranges between 4 and 6 months depending on the patient, the home management of the prosthesis and possible radiation therapy, etc. [1]. In this regard, a 2017 retrospective study analyzed the factors that can affect the average life of the VP. The study found that the type of surgery (total laryngectomy with or without pharyngectomy), the sub-glottic extension, and TNM stage of the tumor do not change statistically significantly device life [2]. A significant role has been identified in radiation therapy with median device life of 59 days for patients undergoing RT and 66 days without RT. The most credited hypothesis believes that postradiation xerostomia may facilitate bacterial and fungal infections, usually counteracted by the antimicrobial action of saliva, resulting in reduced VP life span. On the contrary, other studies found no statistically significant difference in mean VP life between patients undergoing adjuvant RT and patients who have not received postlaryngectomy RT [3, 4].

Another factor that can affect device duration is timing of TEP: median device life of 63 days in case of primary TEP and 54 days in case of secondary TEP. Moreover, indwelling voice prostheses have an average life longer than non-indwelling ones [5]. The routine use of Heat and Moisture Exchanger (HME) correlates to a longer life of the voice prosthesis. Indeed, acting as a barrier, HME allows to keep the tracheostoma and VP cleaner and acting as a humidifier, it reduces the risk of crusting in the trachea and VP [3]. One of the most frequent causes of replacement of the speech prosthesis is the *Candida albicans* (*C. albicans*) colonization, responsible for trans-prosthetic leakage. In their study, Yenigun et al. have reported that fungal colonization significantly reduces average life of voice prosthesis [6].

So, when the VP is no longer working and a peri- or trans-prosthetic leakage is detected, VP replacement should be performed.

5.2   Pre-operative Evaluation

Before replacing the VP, the condition of the tracheostoma, tracheoesophageal fistula, VP, and the presence of indication to its replacement should be assessed. Indeed, it is appropriate to consider the possible peri- or trans-prosthetic leakage and its cause (biofilm clogging the valve, too long prosthesis, dislocation of the VP, etc.), possible infections or granulations, or changes of the tracheostoma. In our clinical practice, using the flexible laryngoscopy, we evaluate the conditions of the esophagus to look for a possible infection of its mucosa (Fig. 5.1), pressure injuries as well as to assess the condition of the esophageal flange of the VP.

Based on the above factors, the type of prosthesis and the mode of replacement are established.

Fig. 5.1 Esophageal candidiasis

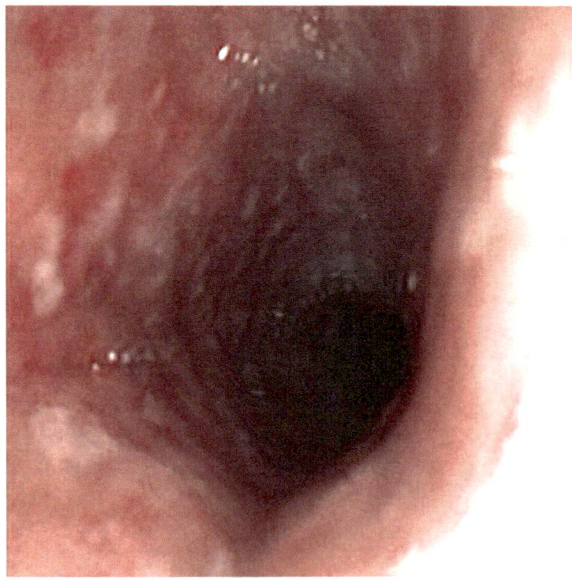

5.3   Voice Prosthesis Replacement Set

In order to perform the replacement of the VP, it is advisable to get some sterile surgical tools (Fig. 5.2):

- Suction tube to aspirate saliva and secretions from tracheoesophageal fistula and tracheostoma during the replacement.
- No. 2–3 angled klemmer forceps to grip the tracheal flange and extract the VP.
- Scissors to cut the retention strap.
- Local anesthetic spray (lidocaine spray 10 g/100 mL for mucosa).
- Length measuring device.
- Shunt dilators (Fig. 5.3).

NB anatomical clamps should be used to avoid damaging the prosthesis and/or damaging the tracheal mucosa during the procedure.

Fig. 5.2 Instrumental set

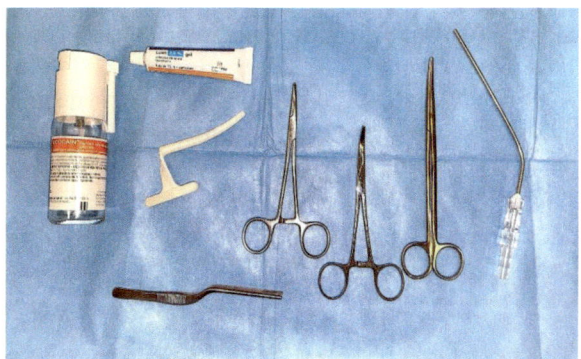

Fig. 5.3 Shunt dilators: Blom-Singer® (**a**) and Provox® (**b**)

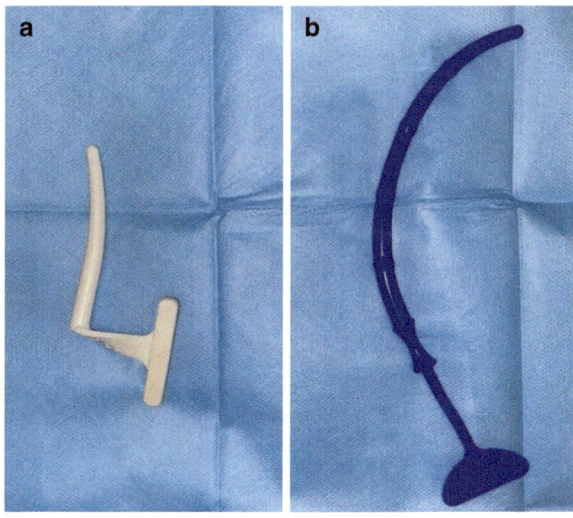

5.4   Preparation of the Patients

Replacement of the speech prosthesis is performed on an outpatient basis under local anesthesia. Indeed, in our clinical practice, local anesthetic spray (lidocaine spray 10 g/100 mL for mucosa) is applied in oropharynx and trachea to minimize the cough reflex and patient discomfort during the procedure.

5.5   Method of VP Replacement

The replacement of the VP can be performed in two ways: anterograde and retrograde. The latter procedure is carried out in special cases where the replacement through the anterograde way would be difficult, e.g., narrow stoma and low TEP. Moreover, retrograde replacement mode is prerogative Provox™ voice prosthesis.

5.5.1   Anterograde Replacement Mode

After removing the VP, the shunt dilator is inserted into the tracheoesophageal fistula. Subsequently, the voice prosthesis shall be inserted from the tracheal side to the esophageal one (Figs. 5.4, 5.5 and 5.6).

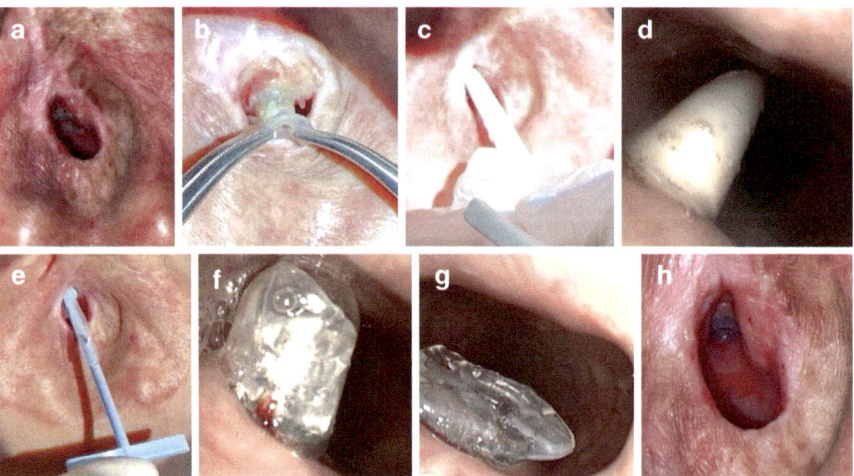

Fig. 5.4 Anterograde replacement of Blom-Singer® voice prosthesis: prosthesis to be replaced (**a**), prosthesis removal (**b**), introduction of dilator, tracheal view (**c**), and esophageal view (**d**), introduction on inserter (**e**), gel cap with prosthesis inside (esophageal view), (**f**) replaced prosthesis after gel cap dissolving (esophageal view) (**g**), prosthesis in situ (**h**)

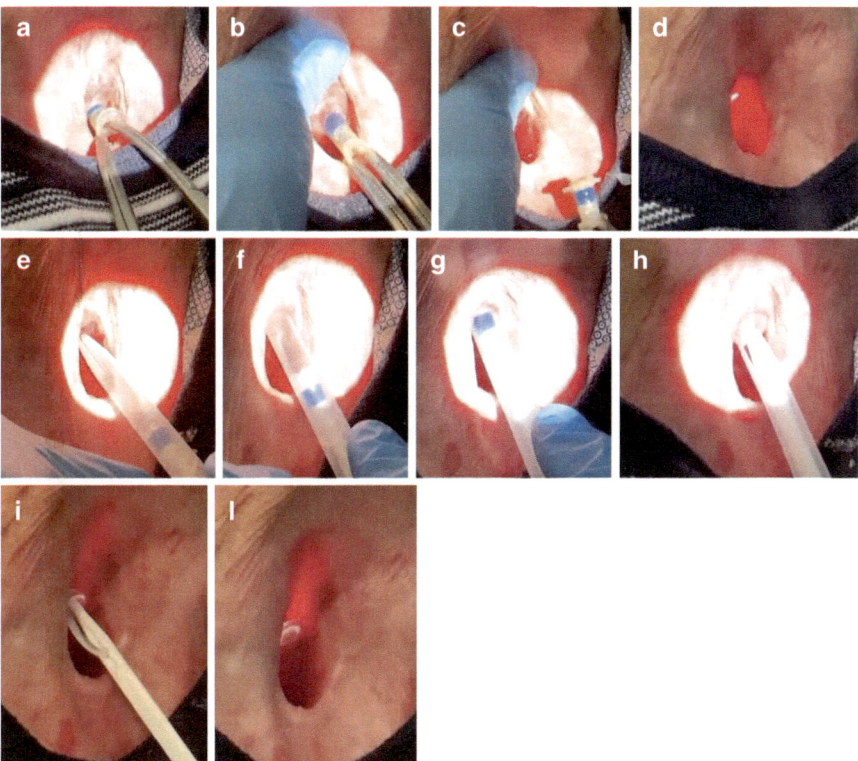

Fig. 5.5 Anterograde replacement of Provox® voice prosthesis (tracheal view): removal of prosthesis (**a–c**), fistula (**d**), introduction of smart inserter (**e–g**), positioning of prosthesis (**h, i**) replaced prosthesis (**l**)

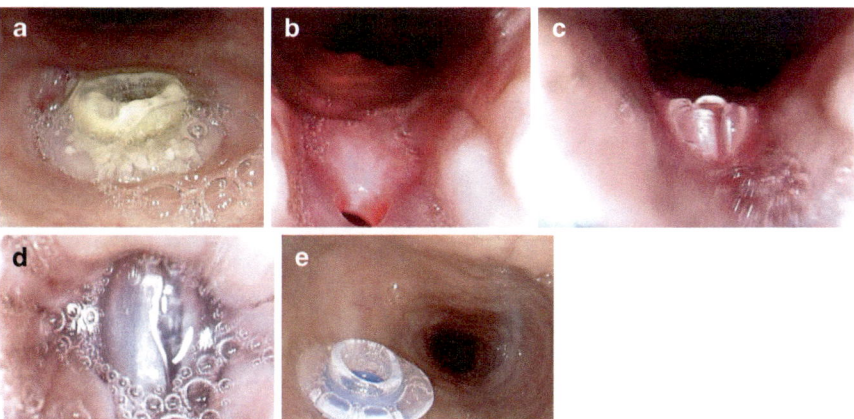

Fig. 5.6 Anterograde replacement of Provox® voice prosthesis (esophageal view): prosthesis to be replaced (**a**), fistula (**b**), introduction of smart inserter (**c, d**), replaced prosthesis (**e**)

5.5.2   Retrograde Replacement Mode

Retrograde replacement involves the use of a guide wire which is passed through the valve of the damaged VP, from the trachea to the esophageal lumen, to reach the pharynx and finally be recovered from the oral cavity. The new VP is fixed on the tip of the guide wire. The tracheal flange of the old VP is grabbed by a curved klemmer and the VP is removed. Then, the end of the wire is retracted so that the attached new VP reaches the esophagus and then the TEP. Pulling further the wire, the prosthesis will be positioned correctly in the fistula [7] (Figs. 5.7 and 5.8).

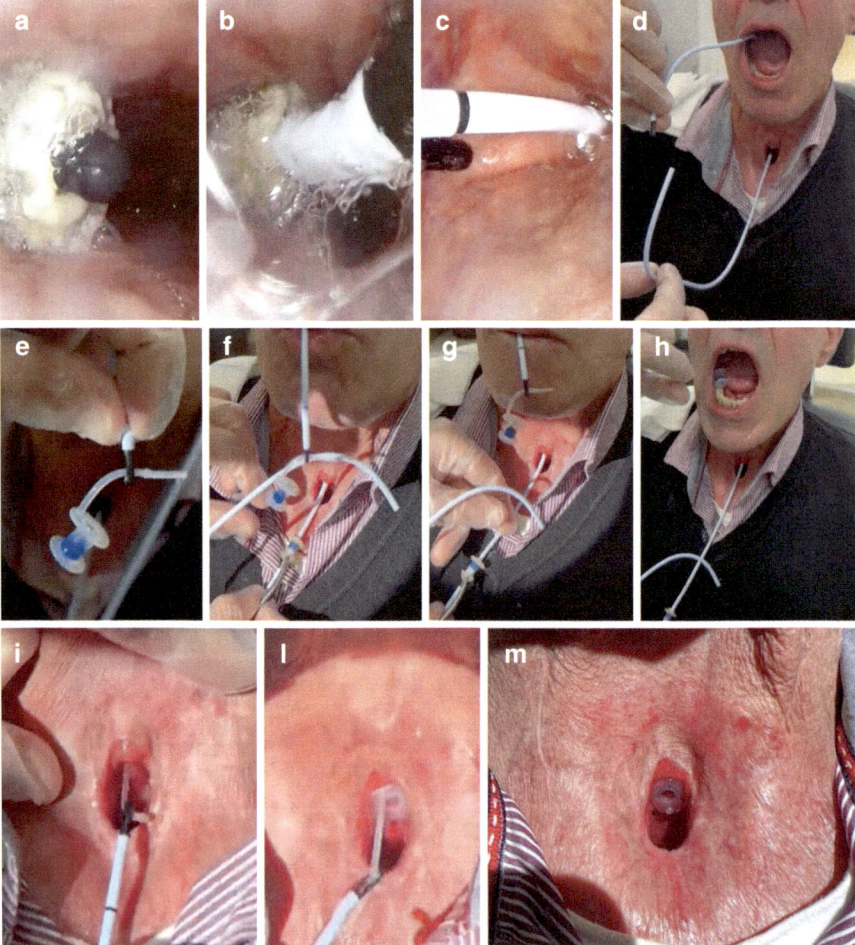

Fig. 5.7   Retrograde replacement of Provox® voice prosthesis: insertion of guide wire through the prosthesis (**a**, **b**), progression of guide wire in hypopharynx (**c**), exiting of guide wire from the mouth (**d**), attachment of prosthesis to the guide wire (**e**), simultaneous extraction and introduction of prosthesis (**f–h**), positioning of new prosthesis (**i**, **l**), replaced prosthesis (**m**)

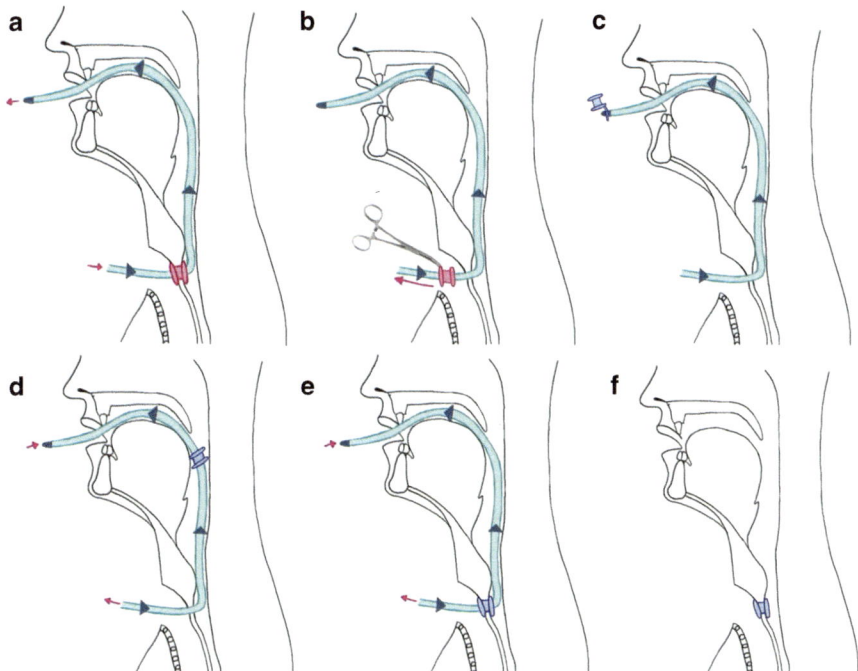

Fig. 5.8 Schematic view of retrograde replacement of Provox® voice prosthesis: insertion of guide wire through the prosthesis and its exiting from the mouth (**a**), extraction of prosthesis (**b**), attachment of new prosthesis to the guide wire (**c**), simultaneous extraction and introduction of prosthesis (**d**), positioning of new prosthesis (**e**), replaced prosthesis (**f**) [with courtesy from Dr. Barbara Verro]

5.6   Final Check

Once the procedure is completed, if deemed necessary, the correct positioning of the esophageal flange of VP is checked endoscopically and the continence of the prosthesis by drinking water and the correct phonation through the prosthesis are assessed.

Declaration by Authors Figures are original and free from copyright issues.

References

1. Hancock KL, Lawson NR, Ward EC. Device life of the Provox Vega voice prosthesis. Eur Arch Otorhinolaryngol. 2013;270(4):1447–53. https://doi.org/10.1007/s00405-012-2154-9.
2. Gitomer SA, Hutcheson KA, Christianson BL, Samuelson MB, Barringer DA, Roberts DB, Hessel AC, Weber RS, Lewin JS, Zafereo ME. Influence of timing, radiation, and reconstruc-

tion on complications and speech outcomes with tracheoesophageal puncture. Head Neck. 2016;38(12):1765–71. https://doi.org/10.1002/hed.24529.
3. Pribuišis K, Pašvenskaitė A, Liutkevičius V, Pajėdienė G, Gaučė G, Uloza V. Factors affecting the lifetime of third-generation voice prosthesis after total laryngectomy. J Voice. 2022;22:27. https://doi.org/10.1016/j.jvoice.2022.01.027. Epub ahead of print.
4. Krishnamurthy A, Khwajamohiuddin S. Analysis of factors affecting the longevity of voice prosthesis following total laryngectomy with a review of literature. Indian J Surg Oncol. 2018;9(1):39–45. https://doi.org/10.1007/s13193-017-0700-z. Epub 2017 Sep 6.
5. Lewin JS, Baumgart LM, Barrow MP, Hutcheson KA. Device life of the tracheoesophageal voice prosthesis revisited. JAMA Otolaryngol Head Neck Surg. 2017;143(1):65–71. https://doi.org/10.1001/jamaoto.2016.2771.
6. Yenigun A, Eren SB, Ozkul MH, Tugrul S, Meric A. Factors influencing the longevity and replacement frequency of Provox voice prostheses. Singap Med J. 2015;56(11):632–6. https://doi.org/10.11622/smedj.2015173.
7. Hilgers FJ, Schouwenburg PF. A new low-resistance, self-retaining prosthesis (Provox) for voice rehabilitation after total laryngectomy. Laryngoscope. 1990;100(11):1202–7. https://doi.org/10.1288/00005537-199011000-00014.

Rehabilitation After Total Laryngectomy

6

6.1 Introduction

Rehabilitation is the "third phase" of the treatment process, in laryngeal carcinoma with total organ removal, subsequent and complementary to the preventive and diagnostic-curative ones.

A patient who receives total laryngectomy surgery is undoubtedly a patient who needs proper rehabilitation [1, 2].

The loss of the larynx organ involves, in fact, the loss of certain functions that can only be replaced, modified, readjusted only through a correct and complete medical rehabilitation.

The skills of certain health professions (speech therapist, physiotherapist, psychotherapist) are fundamental to this process [3, 4]. These professionals, through pre-surgery counseling, know the patient and his or her peculiarities, so they are able to inform him or her, of his respiratory, phonatory, and olfactory recovery potential, and can assist the clinical diagnosis made by the surgeon (even before the surgical act itself) [5].

The opportunity to provide the correct information on the potential recovery of some functions that will be lost as a result of surgery, is a fundamental step to support and prepare the patient psychologically for the post-surgical pathway that he or she will undertake; also taking into consideration that he or she is already strongly stressed, in both psychological and emotional ways, precisely because the communication of the carcinoma diagnosis. Experience show that it is almost always of great help and psychological support to have a meeting, prior to surgery, between the newly diagnosed patient and another patient, who has been operated before and has already achieved excellent levels of rehabilitation. Such encounters are of great help because they make the patient realize that, with the necessary efforts, he or she can be recovered to a "normal life."

Today, it can be considered that the group of therapists involved in the rehabilitation can also fully include so-called volunteer patients (usually organized in

C. Saraniti et al., *Voice Prosthesis in Total Laryngectomized Patients*, https://doi.org/10.1007/978-3-031-29654-3_6

associations) who work together with them for all the support and help that their example and experience can provide [6].

6.2   Respiratory and Pulmonary Rehabilitation

With the complete removal of the larynx organ for oncological reasons (so-called total laryngectomy), the surgeon is forced to separate the upper airways (nose, mouth, nasopharynx) and the lower airways (trachea, bronchus, lungs) though a permanent tracheostomy, which attaches the trachea to the skin and connects the latter directly with the external environment, thus enabling breathing.

In view of this surgical event, the patient loses the respiratory function of the so-called upper airways, with serious repercussions in terms of "purification," "warming," and "humidification" of inhaled air.

Physiological breathing, through the nose, conveys the air inhaled from the external environment (usually at a temperature of around 22 °C and a relative humidity of 40%) into the nasal passages where it is heated (until it reaches 29 °C) and humidified (humidity rises to 70%). This process, once past the nasal cavities, continues all the way from the external air to the lungs (Fig. 6.1) [7].

In fact, once past the larynx organ, at the level of the subglottis, the air temperature will reach 32 °C with 100% relative humidity; instead, once reached the lungs, air temperature will be around 36 °C (equivalent to body temperature). Unfortunately, this does not happen when breathing occurs through tracheostomy. In that case, incoming air will have a temperature around 22 °C and will reach the lower airways at a temperature of 27–28 °C, with a relative humidity of 50%. Studies over the last 20 years show that, when this happens, the cold, slightly moist air causes an

Fig. 6.1 Lower respiratory tract anatomy [with courtesy from Dr. Barbara Verro]

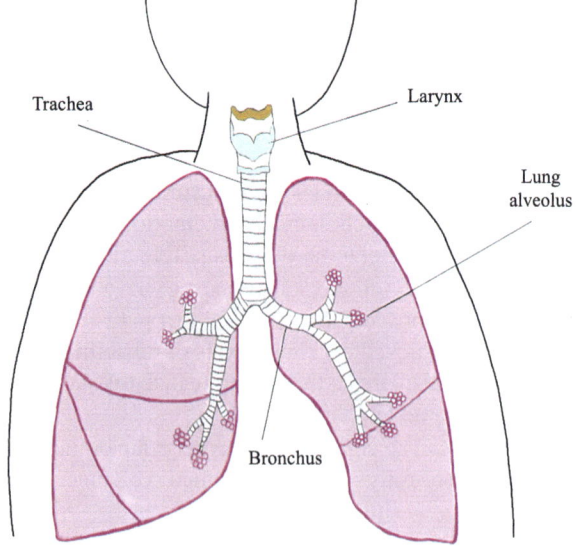

Trachea

Larynx

Lung alveolus

Bronchus

alteration in muco-ciliary activity, resulting in a progressive slowdown in its movement, up to a complete stop; with inevitable accumulation of secretions and mucus in the tracheo-bronchial walls [8, 9]. This inactivity of "mucociliary clearance" results in an inability to filter and protect against viruses, bacteria, and particles such as allergens, pollen, and dust, with consequent accumulation of these particles in the lower airways, exposing the subject to the risk of developing recurrent respiratory infections. Precisely the worst side effect of post-total laryngectomy complained of by patients, it is excessive mucus production (which, among other things, severely limits their social relationships). They complain of respiratory symptoms that inevitably translate into sleep disturbances, fatigue, shortness of breath, poor vocal quality, in an overall serious deterioration of the patient's quality of life [10].

For the speech therapist, taking care of a laryngectomised patient means: preparatory work on the patient's acceptance of the tracheostomy, the explanation of simplified instructions to be used in order to fully understand the new respiration and the use of the technical aids (medical devices), fundamental to restoring respiration as similar as possible to the physiological one [10].

With regard to breathing aids, the most important are artificial noses or Heat and Moisture Exchanger (HME) filters.

These perform three fundamental functions [11, 12]:

– Particle filtration, bringing in cleaner air.
– Humidification and warming of the incoming air, with restoration of muco-ciliary activity and progressive reduction of dry mucus deposited in the lower respiratory tract. Warm, moist air dissolves mucus and prevents it from being deposited for a long time. The exchange of heat and moisture occurs thanks to the retention of water by the filter, which consists of a sponge placed inside a plastic housing [13].
– Partial restoration of respiratory resistance, with reactivation of the respiratory muscles.

The protocol for the use of the HME filter includes its application in the immediate post-operative period. These filters can be attached to rigid tracheostomy cannulae, to soft silicone cannulae, and finally to a so-called peristomal patch. These aids have a 15 mm, 22 mm, or 23 mm slot precisely for the application of the HME filter. The therapist's aim is to prevent "free tracheostomy" breathing, which leads the patient to become accustomed to incorrect breathing, creating serious airway problems. In addition, a patient who is not used to aids will have difficulty adapting to breathing with an HME filter (in our experience, patients who have not been correctly looked after from the start suffer from suffocation and breathing difficulties when switching to the correct aid, also due to a debilitation of the diaphragmatic muscles as a result of previous breathing without natural inspiratory resistance). To help the therapist dealing with patients who have not used anything to support the breathing process for a longer or shorter period, there are two types of HME filters which differ in the type of filter weave (narrow-meshed or wide-meshed) and thus in the type of inspiratory resistance applied. In these cases, the protocol includes the

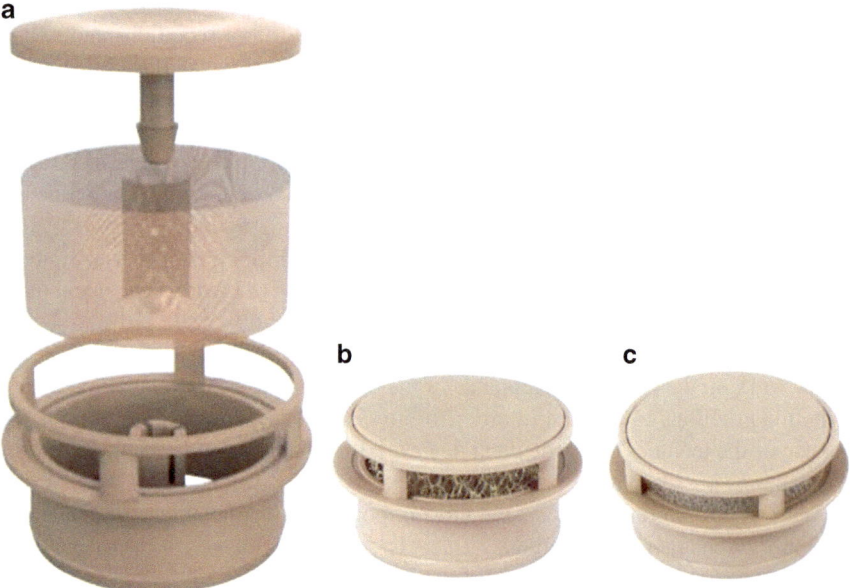

Fig. 6.2 Types of Heat and Moisture Exchanger (HME) filters: inner structure of filter (**a**), filters with a large-mesh sponge (**b**) and with a narrow-mesh sponge (**c**)

initial use of the lowest breathing resistance filter, with a large-mesh sponge, to gradually proceed with the replacement with a higher breathing resistance filter, with a narrow-mesh sponge. The latter can guarantee the restoration of near-physiological nasal breathing [8] (Fig. 6.2). The wide-mesh filter is also suitable for athletes, who need frequent air exchanges with less respiratory resistance during physical activity. However, it has been proved that all laryngectomised patients, regardless the mode of vocal function's restoration, should use the filters continuously 24/7 [14]. Due to their low profile, unobtrusive design, such aids are usually well tolerated. Furthermore, the use of such HME filters is specifically (but not exclusively) designed for patients who have had a phonatory prosthesis implanted. In fact, they can activate an additional function of such filters, which, thanks to their "button" shape with slight digital pressure, closes the air flow in exhalation and thereby facilitates the expiratory thrust in the direction of the phonatory prosthesis and thus aids phonation itself.

The HME filter creates short- and long-term benefits [15]:

- Short-term benefits:
  - Restoration of physiological respiratory resistance.
  - In patients using this aid, a reactivation of the mucosal cilia is observed sometime after the operation, with an initial increase in expectoration of mucus and elimination of accumulated mucus.
  - In general, better oxygenation leads to greater general well-being.

- Long-term benefits:
  - General improvement in lung function, with reduced expectoration of mucus.
  - A restoration of mucociliary activity is observed in patients adopting this aid some time after the surgery.
  - Reduced exposure to infectious respiratory diseases.
  - Improved sleep quality, reduced anxiety, character susceptibility and depression, related to the discomfort of overproduction of mucus.
  - Improved phonation, with adequate intelligibility of the voice, in the absence of noise from the tracheostomy [16].

In terms of restoring the physiological breathing of the upper respiratory tract, the HME filter, although not yet able to achieve results that are completely comparable on the physiological ones, in terms of temperature and humidity increase, is able to guarantee an increase in relative temperature from 27–28 °C to 29–30 °C and relative humidity from 50 to 70%. As already mentioned, HME filters can be anchored to tracheostomy cannulas or peristomal adhesive, in accordance with a variety of needs. Moreover, there are numerous types of adhesives on the market in order to be able to meet the different needs of patients, especially in view of the physiological characteristics and conformation of the peristomal skin and the tracheostomy itself (Fig. 6.3).

In addition, these peristomal adhesives are also designed for the use of additional aids, besides HME filters, such as:

- Automatic valve for hands-free phonation.
- Shower device.
- Some types of silicone tracheostomic cannulae that do not have fastening straps (Fig. 6.4).

Fig. 6.3 HME filters positioned in to peristomal adhesive

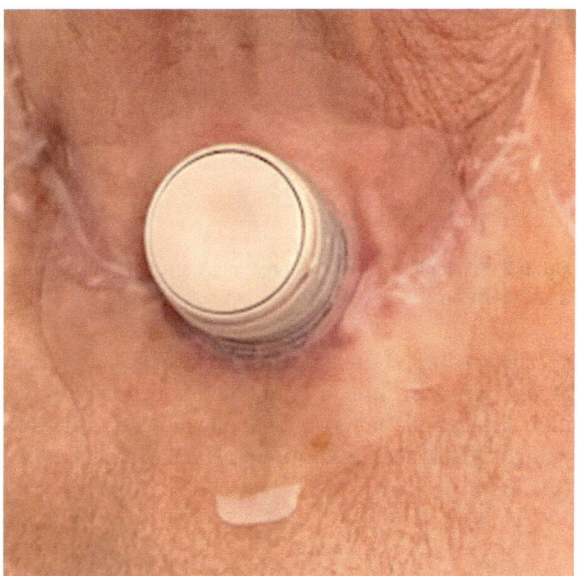

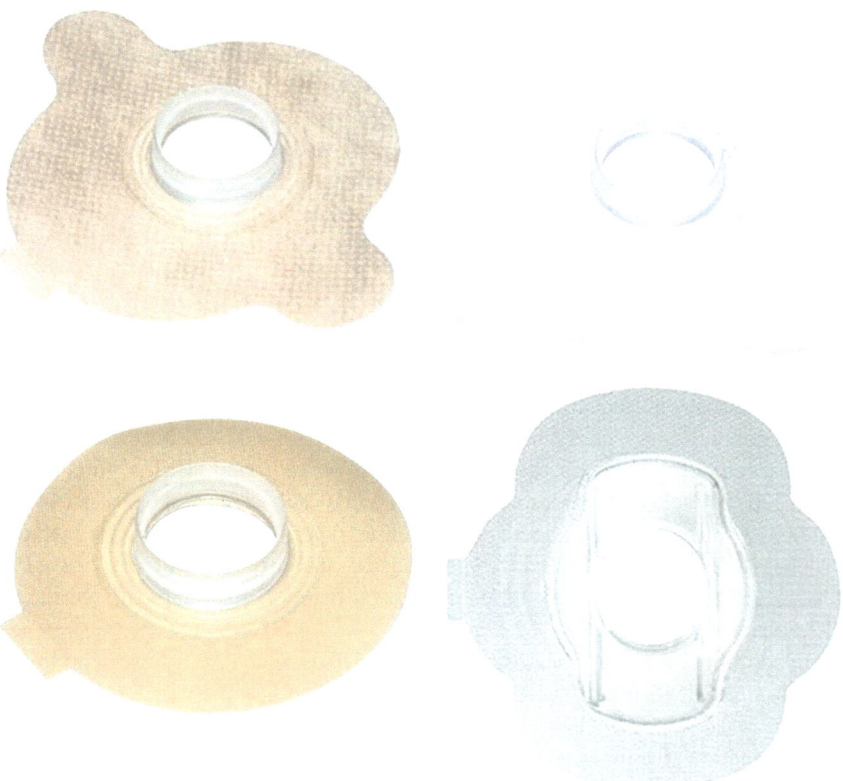

Fig. 6.4 Different types of peristomal adhesives

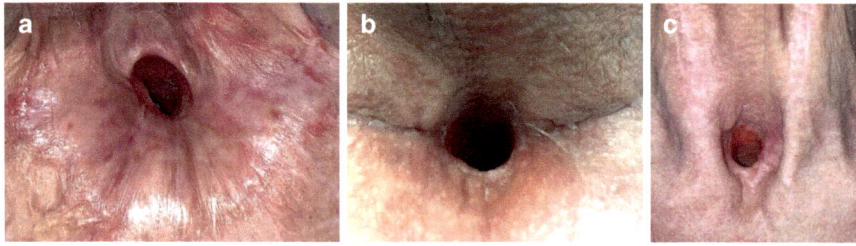

Fig. 6.5 Examples of tracheostoma: neck after radiotherapy (**a**), flat tracheostoma (**b**), and deep tracheostoma (**c**)

These adhesives may also vary in material type and shape. The choice of one model of plaster instead of another, which is closely discussed with the clinician, must achieve the purpose of application for a duration of 24–48 h, guaranteeing optimal adherence. Below are practical examples of the use and choice of a plaster (Fig. 6.5):

- Neck after radiotherapy: plaster with hydrogel.
- Presence of the sternal heads of the SCMD: plaster with rigid base.
- Small, sunken tracheostomy: rigid support.
- Excessive sweating: water-repellent plaster with high adhesive power.

Most plasters are made of hypoallergenic materials (ethylene butyl acrylate and polyethylene) that respect the peristomal skin while providing flexibility and resistance. There are hydrocolloid (water and colloid) adhesives, which are suitable for sensitive and/or radio-treated skin. After making the selection of the plaster, based on the material and type, the size and shape are evaluated and the one considered most suitable for the patient is chosen (e.g., a round, oval or oval extralarge-XL plaster). The above-mentioned plasters are applied to the peristomal skin by means of special adhesives with which they are impregnated. In order, however, to ensure a better daily hold, additional aids such as wipes with different functions can be used:

- Preparation of the skin, protecting it from irritation and improving the adhesion of the adhesive.
- The atraumatic removal of the adhesive, with the melting of its glue.
- Cleansing of the skin to remove peristomal glue residue from the removed adhesive.

Having started the correct protocol of using the HME filter, the patient can undertake, with the help of the speech therapist, relaxation training of the cervical and scapulohumeral musculature, continuing with linguo-occus-facial exercises aimed at reactivating the vocal tract. These exercises are fundamental for achieving adequate phonation with the use of the phonatory prosthesis.

6.2.1 Muscle and Pragmatic Relaxation Exercises

- Massage the scar on the neck (Fig. 6.6). The massage can be performed by the patient or caregiver.
- Pull the scar gently to stretch it and make it soft.

  Sitting, upright torso, head tilt:

- Toward the right shoulder.
- Back.
- Toward the left shoulder.
- Forward on the chest.
- Making a full circle (Fig. 6.7).

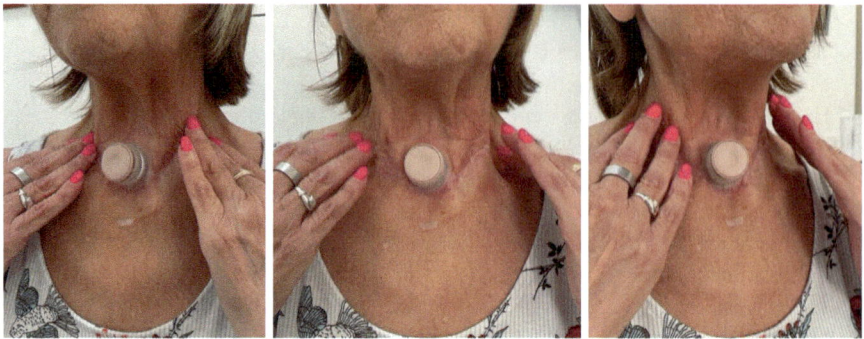

Fig. 6.6 Massage of the neck scar

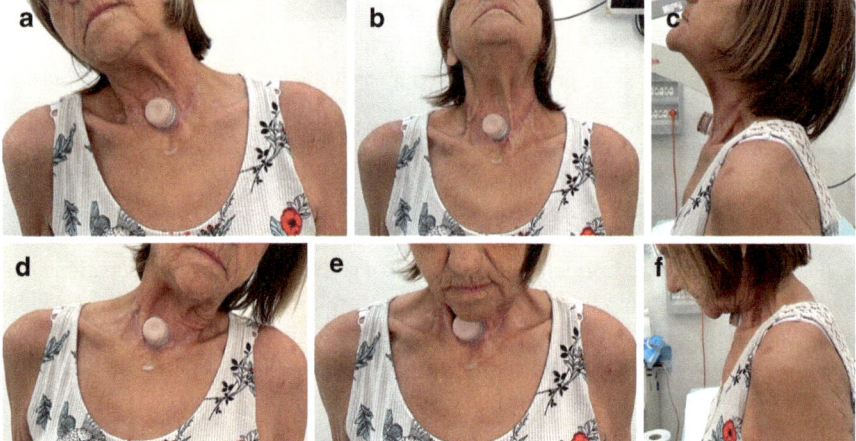

Fig. 6.7 Head tilt toward the right shoulder (**a**), back (**b, c**), toward the left shoulder (**d**), forward on the chest (**e, f**)

All movements must be performed very slowly.
For the neck muscles:

– Open and close your mouth as much as you can (Fig. 6.8).
– Pull the tongue out as far as possible and retract it (Fig. 6.8).
– Making "faces" (Fig. 6.8).
– Hold these positions for a few seconds.
– Lift and lower the shoulders as much as possible (Fig. 6.9).
– Keep your arms relaxed along your body.
– Interlock your fingers and extend your arms forward.
– Turn your palms out.

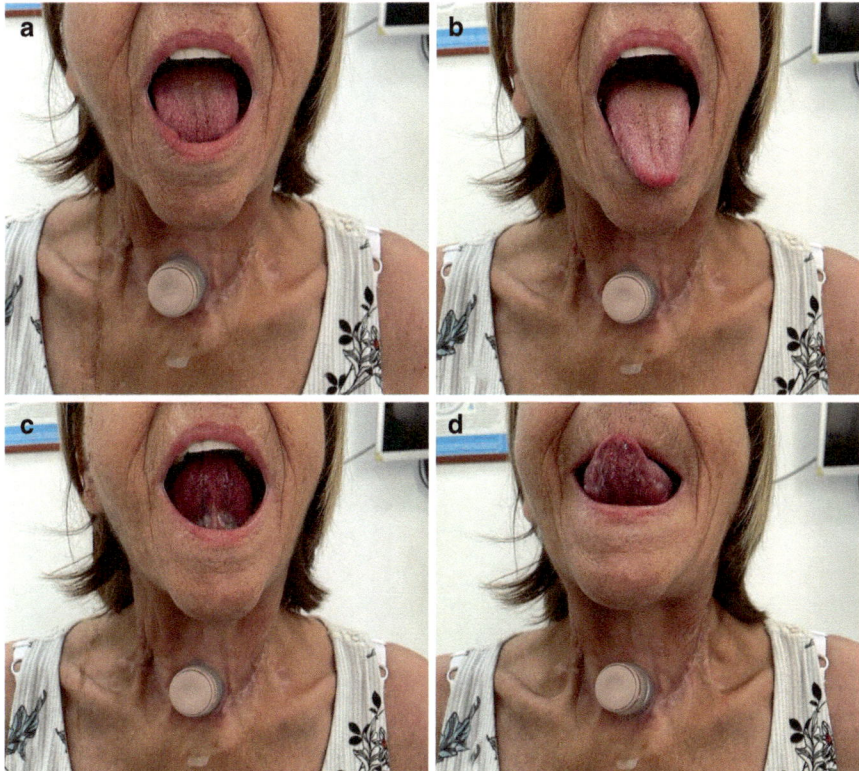

Fig. 6.8 Open and close your mouth as much as you can (**a**); pull the tongue out as far as possible and retract it (**b, c**); making "faces" (**d**)

- Extend your arms (Fig. 6.10).
- Keep your arms extended above your head.
- With the right hand grasp the left hand and pull the arm slowly (Fig. 6.10), grasp your right hand and repeat the same exercise.
- Fingers interlaced behind the nape of the neck. Bring the elbows out while keeping the torso and head well aligned.
- Bring your right hand to your left shoulder.
- Rest your left hand on your right elbow.
- Gently push the elbow toward the left shoulder, perform the same exercise on the other side.

In a sitting position, grasp the stick by the ends, keeping your arms straight in front of your body:

Fig. 6.9 Lift and lower
the shoulders as much as
possible

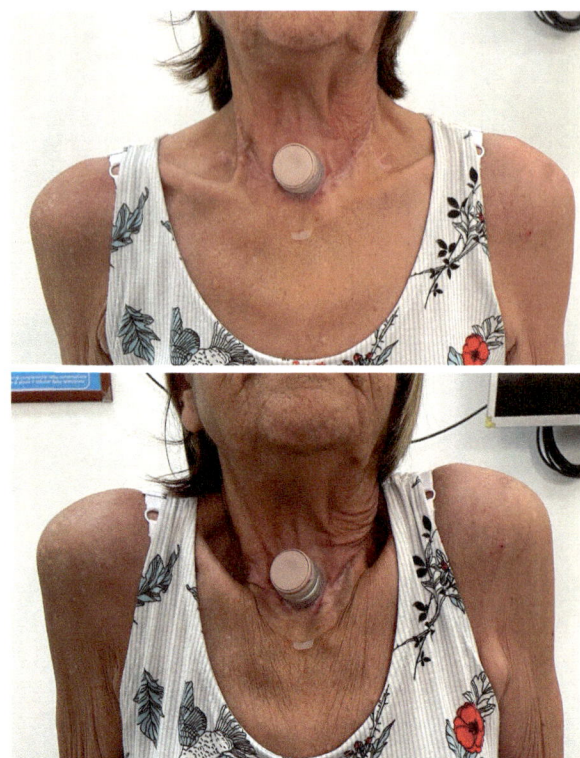

– Move the stick as far and as close to the body as you can.
– Bring the stick to the right and then to the left following the movement.
– Carry the stick behind your back with your palms facing upwards.
– Move the stick upwards away from the body while keeping the elbows extended
  and without reclining the torso forward.

The exercises must be performed daily (each session must be of short duration) with constancy and at levels of progressive difficulty, gradually dosing the effort and without overdoing it. These exercises are proposed in speech therapy sessions, as early as the tenth post-surgery day, both in subjects implanted with a phonatory prosthesis and in those without a prosthesis (or for whom it has been decided to implant it afterwards). The aim of the exercises is, in fact, to improve agility in movements that have become difficult as a result of compromised nerve and muscle structures. The hypomobility of the post-surgery neck and oral cavity immediately after surgery also necessitates daily muscle stretching once the surgical wounds have been recovered.

The prosthetised patient will also work on cost-diaphragmatic breathing and pneumo-phonic coordination (Fig. 6.11).

Fig. 6.10 Extend your
arms (**a**, **b**), with the right
hand grasp the left hand
and pull the arm slowly (**c**)

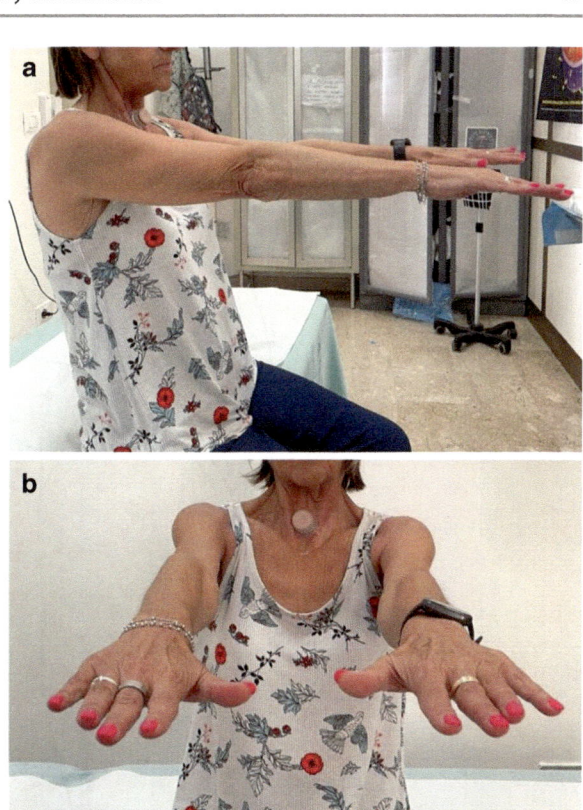

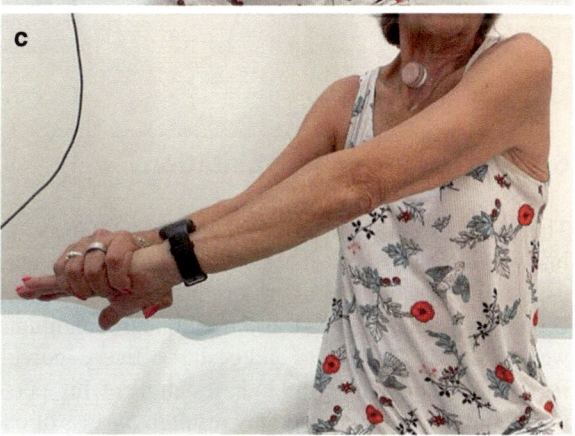

Fig. 6.11 Costal breathing
(**a**); abdominal breathing
(**b**) [with courtesy from Dr.
Barbara Verro]

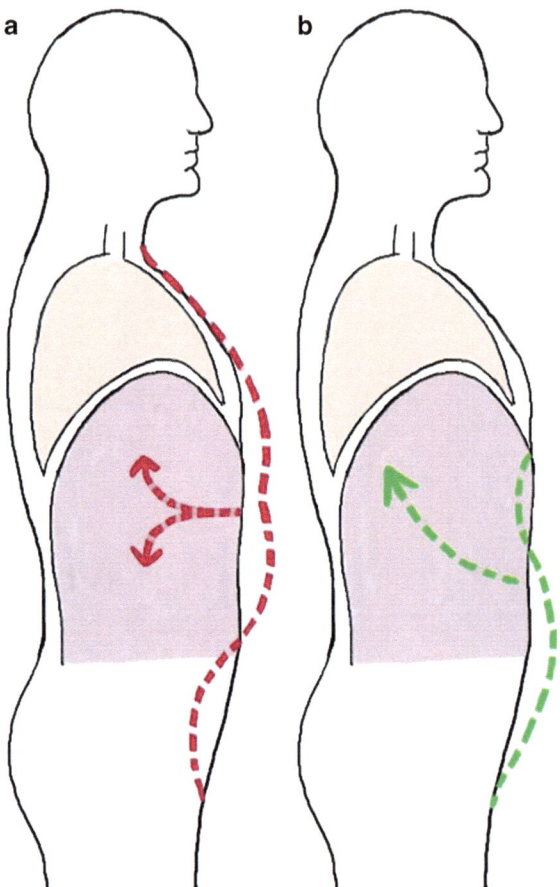

6.3   Phonatory Rehabilitation

The voice has always been called the mirror of the soul. Every emotion is translated
into words through our voice, and nothing can be concealed. The voice speaks about
us, it tells the world about our origins, our experiences, and our history. Losing it,
becomes a rather dramatic event, although communication can continue through
writing, the use of mimics and gestures. Every individual deprived of his voice is,
inevitably, deprived of the manifestation of his personality [17]. Unfortunately,
undergoing a total laryngectomy result in the loss of one's voice and, with it, part of
one's "self," which is difficult to recover, even with a vicarious voice. Today, sci-
ence and technology, gifted us with tools suitable for phonatory recovery, which, for
the most part, lead to the phonatory prosthesis implant. Often, however, it is necessary to work on the acceptance of the new voice. This acceptance process is driven,
only in part, by the need to recover one's personality. In most cases, the desire to

return to speaking must be supported by a process that facilitates the psychological acceptance of the new voice and, at the same time, teaches the use of the prosthesis to achieve the best possible phonatory performance [18]. The motivation to speak again, even if with a new voice, sometimes unpleasant to listen for those who are not used to dialogue with a prosthetised subject, is the key element, the machine that moves everything, without it the patient could never return to speaking [19, 20]. It often happens to encounter subjects who are not very talkative, taciturn. They spoke little even before the operation, so all the difficulties they may encounter after total laryngectomy lead them to unwillingness to get involved in acquiring their new voice. Conversely, many total laryngectomy patients, deprived of their voice (often an indispensable means for the continuation of their working career, as well as for the continuation of interpersonal relationships) make their prosthetic voice the only lifeline from an otherwise inevitable social isolation. Reaffirming the possibility of being able to communicate in writing or by taking advantage of new technologies (multimedia apps, etc...), it is only with the voice that one recovers the true identity lost under the surgical knife, after the removal of the larynx and thus of the vocal cords.

6.3.1 Phonatory Rehabilitation Sessions

The laryngectomized patient uses the phonatory prothesis, causing a nullification of the expiratory air outflow, pushing the air to seek a different exit route. The tracheoesophageal prosthesis, on the other hand, placed into the esophagus, vibrates the cricopharyngeal tract (called, for this reason, the "neolarynx") [21].

Phonatory rehabilitation varies with respect to the time of implantation of the phonatory prosthesis.

6.3.1.1 Post-operative Training in Primary

1. Pneumo-phonic and oculo-manual co-ordination for correct typing of the tracheostomy. This must be approached, in the first instance, without the use of the button filter, which in turn is anchored to a cannula or patch. In this way, with total occlusion of the tracheostomy, one works on the acquisition of the gestures that will lead to phonation. By exploiting the patient's working memory, one gets used to phonation by closing the tracheostomy, without any vents and thus possible obstructions due to the presence of the cannula [22] (Fig. 6.12).

2. When the patient has learnt the correct gesture with digital occlusion of the tracheostomy, he/she is instructed to clean the voice prosthesis with a suitable cleaning brush and to place the stomatal plaster and the HME filter. It is important to observe the time required to fix the glue of the plaster to the tracheostomy, to prevent it from coming off at the first occlusion stress of the tracheostomy, during phonation. It only takes about 5 min, and the patient is ready to speak (Fig. 6.13).

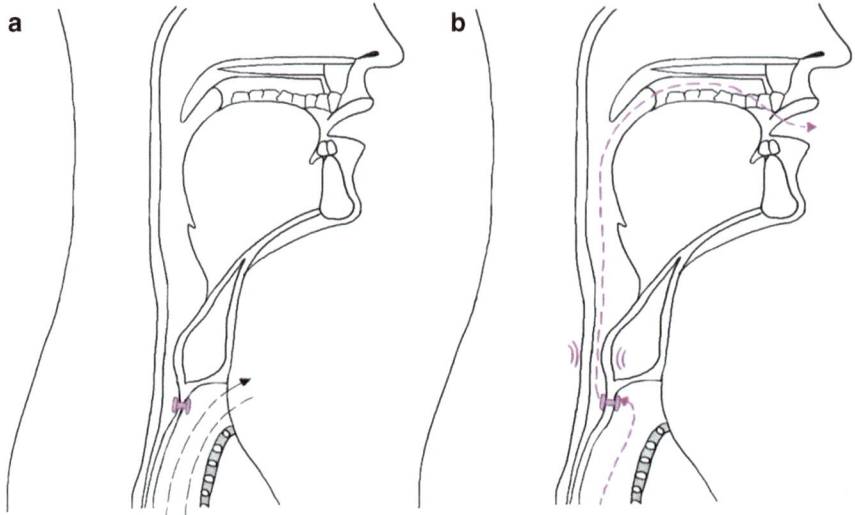

Fig. 6.12 Patient with voice prosthesis: breathing (**a**); phonation (**b**) [with courtesy from Dr. Barbara Verro]

Fig. 6.13 Cleaning the voice prosthesis with a suitable cleaning brush

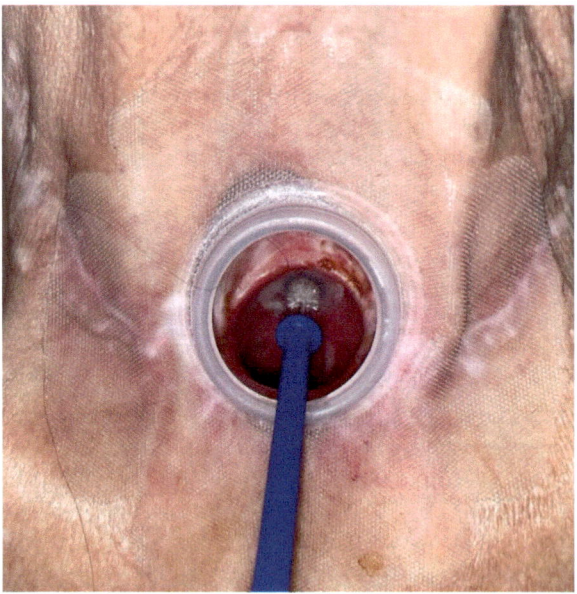

3. The sequence of exercises varies according to the passing of the first phonatory tests, which are generally vocalisations of the letter "A" for a prolonged time. After passing the test and evaluating the cricopharyngeal vibratory tract, we proceed with [23]:

- Automatisms with numbering (numbers from 1 to 10), the months of the year, the days of the week.
- List of bisyllabic words.
- Words related to the personal sphere (names of family members) and greeting formulas.
- Reading of short passages.
- Short sentences on free conversation.
- Guided conversation with questions in the form of an interview.
- Telephone conversation.

6.3.1.2 Post-operative Training in Secondary

The TAUB TEST is considered an excellent preoperative indicator of new tracheo-esophageal entry (hereafter "TE") (Fig. 6.14).

It is essential to enable the patient to hear his new TE voice. The test is conducted with the insertion of a 14 Fr tube, 50 cm long, to be inserted up to the height of the tracheostomy. The other end consists of a plastic ring that can be attached to the stoma patch. The patient has to inhale, close the tracheostomy by blowing air into the cricopharyngeal segment from the caterer, which should vibrate for 8–10 s.

Speech therapy sessions may continue for approximately 1 month after the patient's hospital discharge. Some studies show that five speech therapy sessions may be sufficient to train the patient in the use of the phonatory prosthesis.

Evaluation of improvements in phonation can be based on objective measurements, such as [24]:

- The maximum phonatory time: 4–21 s.
- The number of words in a single vent: 1.14–2.5.
- Voice frequency (Hz) 8–10 [25].

Worldwide literature states that patients with phonatory prostheses are able to say up to 16 words with each breath (definitely an advantage over the 5–7 words in the case of esophageal voice).

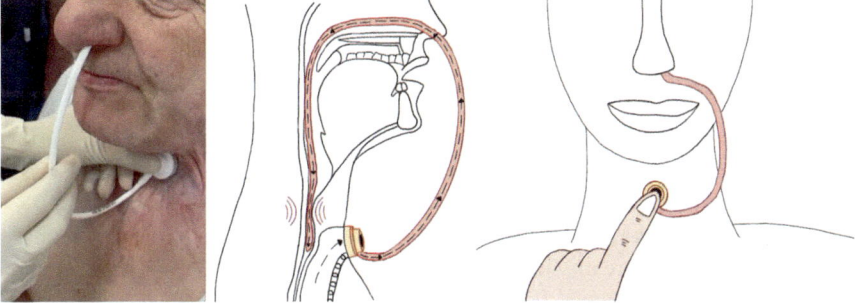

Fig. 6.14 TAUB test [with courtesy from Dr. Barbara Verro]

In addition to examining the phonatory possibilities of the patient in terms of pulmonary bellows, adequate breathing for effective sound emission, other predictive parameters for a correct rehabilitation of the voice and oesophageal speech must be taken into consideration, namely shape of the hypopharyngeal funnel, absence of hypertonicity, extent of the resection of the mucous membrane of the pharynx. In these cases, logopaedic rehabilitation could benefit from parallel medical-surgical treatment in order to improve prosthetic performance [24]. Another study comparing the post-total laryngectomy replacement voice (esophageal voice, tracheoesophageal voice, and laryngophone voice), confirms that the prosthetic voice is the most communicative in terms of lift, economy of production, effectiveness, intelligibility, and reliability in speech [26].

6.3.2   Public Speaking

When a process of phonatory rehabilitation is initiated, the patient is able, within the therapeutic setting, to get involved, to experiment his new voice and to speak without relevant difficulties. But it becomes, almost, a practitioner–patient communication, as if the patient recognises in the speech therapist that figure capable of understanding him/her, who does not judge his/her way of speaking, who does not get upset if he/she has to close a "hole in the neck" in order to speak.

Outside the setting, even the first word spoken to the family member in the waiting room is loaded with anxieties, fears and therefore difficulties. Just as reaching "social" spaces, making a request in a supermarket or post office, are events charged with worries about the judgment of those in front of you. So, one often stops using the phonatory prosthesis when speaking in public, choosing the universal language for all, which is that of gestures. The patient, communicating with gestures, will find it more difficult to make himself understood but will remain convinced that, by doing so, people will ask fewer questions about his communicative state, about that new voice and about his condition.

Bringing the patient to the naturalness of gestures for phonation, to the manual typing of the speech filter, is certainly possible by confrontation, for example, within the framework of his speech therapy sessions, with patients who have already been using the phonatory prosthesis for some time and play a psychological "mirror" role for the acquisition of the confidence that is still lacking.

Often, this dialogue is created within non-hospital contexts, so that over a coffee in a café, the patient can experience the naturalness of someone who has already overcome their fears.

Regarding reintegration into the social environment in which laryngectomised patients live (and, where possible, the resumption of employment), it is undisputed that such patients will have difficulties.

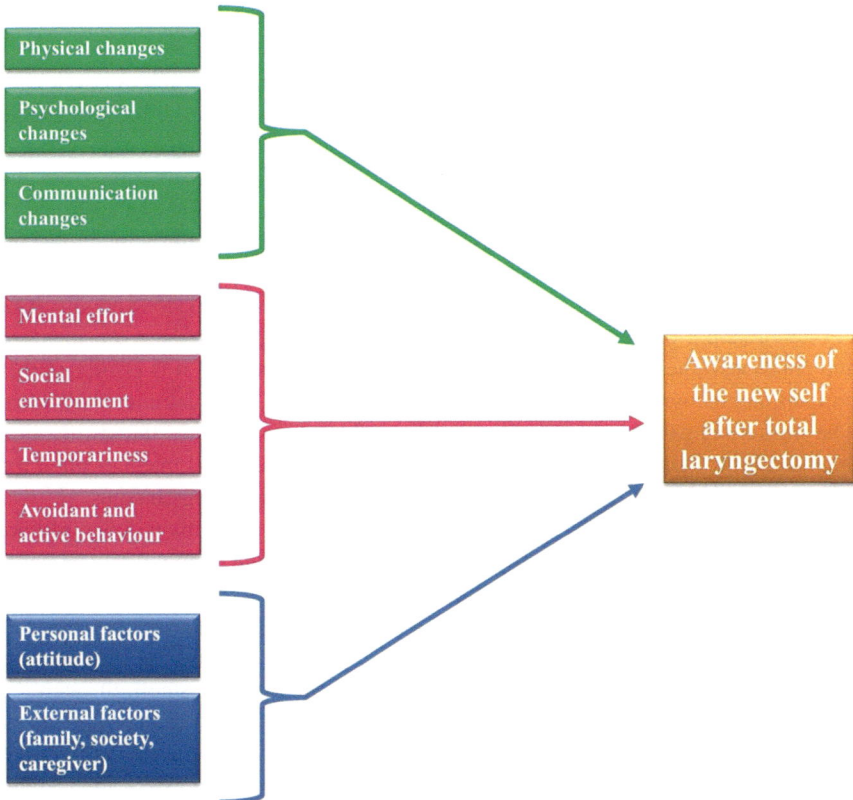

Fig. 6.15 Scheme about the new awareness of the self after total laryngectomy

It can often take up to a year, a time that varies with respect to the possible start of radio-chemotherapy cycles.

It also happens that the patient is unable, for physical and/or psychological reasons, to resume his or her work and is forced, at a relatively young age, to reinvent his or her life [18].

Vocal and speech rehabilitation after placement of the TE prosthesis requires teamwork, ranging from the surgical placement of the prosthesis itself, considered the best alternative for developing communication post total laryngectomy, through rehabilitation conducted in hospital and outpatient treatment lasting up to 1 month. The family entourage and psychological support are fundamental as soon as the diagnosis is communicated but continue to be so especially when the return home implies acceptance of a new body, a new voice and therefore a new life (Fig. 6.15) [27, 28].

6.4   Rehabilitation of the Sense of Smell

Total laryngectomy surgery also implies the loss of the sense of smell (air no longer passes through the mouth and nose and, therefore, the anatomical tract responsible for this sense is skipped) [29].

From a purely anatomical point of view, we know that information from the sense of smell is processed by the *limbic system* (hippocampus and amygdala), which controls emotions, moods, and instincts, and by the *thalamus*, which together with certain areas of the frontal neocortex, is involved in the cognitive interpretation of the olfactory stimulus. In addition, the limbic system and limbic lobe are involved in memorisation processes; what occurs is a mediation process between memory and emotions. These form the basis of the learning process, and it is estimated that humans can recognise thousands of different odours [30]. This explains why when a laryngectomy patient report smelling coffee or his wife's perfume, the justification is given in the memory of that smell. In fact, if the same patient is made to smell the same odours but with the variant of blindfolded eyes, everything changes. He will no longer be able to distinguish wine from coffee, garlic from his wife's perfume. They retain the memory of certain smells, pleasant or not, but cannot really perceive them. Added to this is the danger of not being able to perceive, for example, a gas leak. It therefore seems essential, with a view to their acquiring independence in daily life, to be able to recognise a danger by smell as well. For these reasons, it is always a good idea to start a recovery process for the sense of smell, through the gradual acquisition of suitable techniques and manoeuvres to send air (and therefore odours) back to the olfactory receptors of the nose. According to the study promoted by the *Netherlands Cancer Institute*, there is a technique, based on a manoeuvre known as the NAIM manoeuvre (nasal airflow induction manoeuvre), also known as the *polite yawning* technique [31]. In a speech therapy session, before working on the manoeuvre, the patient is stimulated to smell, assessing the actual activity of his olfactory receptors, with a laryngeal bypass. This is a tube that, connected to the tracheostomy and placed inside the buccal cavity, is able to connect the lower airway with the upper airway. The patient is asked to inhale and exhale through the tube so that the air reaches the nose and allows odours to be smelled. In this way, the patient is able to inhale air again through the nasal cavities; the entry of air into the nasal passages results in the activation of the olfactory epithelium cells. The laryngeal bypass is considered a propaedeutic tool for olfactory rehabilitation and to accustom the patient to a gradual perception of various scented essences.

6.4.1   The NAIM Manoeuvre

The movement that is proposed to the patient is somewhat reminiscent of the movement that every subject performs during a yawn with the mouth open, which is why it is called the "yawning technique," the term "polite" on the other hand refers to the fact that the patient, after constant training, must be able to replicate the proposed movement with the closed mouth, just as a yawn is performed (Fig. 6.16).

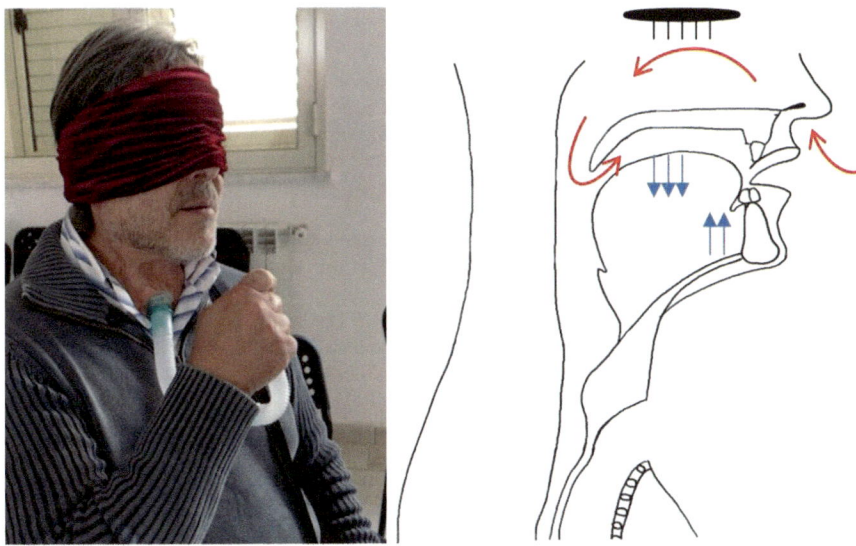

Fig. 6.16 Scheme about the new awareness of the self after total laryngectomy [28]

The processes of which the NAIM manoeuvre is composed are as follows:

- The mandible, thus also the floor of the mouth, is lowered; the mandibular joint rotates, but does not move off its axis.
- At the same time, the tongue body begins to make a movement from the floor of the mouth toward the hard palate.
- Initially, the patient may perform this movement with the mouth open, but once the process is automated, the lips remain closed.
- These movements must be repeated a couple of times and quickly.
- During the execution of the manoeuvre, attention must be paid to the patient's breathing to avoid hyperventilation.

The technique, therefore, is mainly characterized by a rapid movement performed by the tongue which, pressing against the palate, is able to generate pressure inside the oral cavity. This pressure and the consequent airflow generated are transmitted, in the presence of the lowering of the palatine veil, to the nasal cavities, consequently determining an activation of the olfactory cells and allowing the perception of odours.

Having set the manoeuvre, one can proceed with proposing a series of food and non-food fragrances to make the technique tangible in its effectiveness. The patient will need to repeat it several times a day, in conjunction with their main meals or when they feel they can smell odors.

Declaration by Authors Figures are original and free from copyright issues.

References

1. Robertson SM, Yeo JC, Dunnet C, Young D, Mackenzie K. Voice, swallowing, and quality of life after total laryngectomy: results of the west of Scotland laryngectomy audit. Head Neck. 2012;34(1):59–65. https://doi.org/10.1002/hed.21692. Epub 2011 Mar 17.
2. Zenga J, Goldsmith T, Bunting G, Deschler DG. State of the art: rehabilitation of speech and swallowing after total laryngectomy. Oral Oncol. 2018;86:38–47. https://doi.org/10.1016/j.oraloncology.2018.08.023. Epub 2018 Sep 12.
3. Bickford JM, Coveney J, Baker J, Hersh D. Support following total laryngectomy: exploring the concept from different perspectives. Eur J Cancer Care (Engl). 2018;27(3):e12848. https://doi.org/10.1111/ecc.12848. Epub 2018 Apr 19.
4. Parrilla C, Longobardi Y, Paludetti G, Marenda ME, D'Alatri L, Bussu F, Scarano E, Galli J. A 1-year time frame for voice prosthesis management. What should the physician expect? Is it an overrated job? Acta Otorhinolaryngol Ital. 2020;40(4):270–6. https://doi.org/10.14639/0392-100X-N0587. PMID: 33100338; PMCID: PMC7586190.
5. Rosa VM, Fores JML, da Silva EPF, Guterres EO, Marcelino A, Nogueira PC, Baia WRM, Kulcsar MAV. Interdisciplinary interventions in the perioperative rehabilitation of total laryngectomy: an integrative review. Clinics (Sao Paulo). 2018;73(suppl 1):e484s. https://doi.org/10.6061/clinics/2018/e484s.
6. Betlejewski S, Ossowski R, Sinkiewicz A. Rehabilitacja chorych po laryngektomii—wizja a realizacja [rehabilitation after total laryngectomy—vision and realization]. Otolaryngol Pol. 2007;61(3):344–8. https://doi.org/10.1016/S0030-6657(07)70441-9.
7. Keck T, Leiacker R, Heinrich A, Kühnemann S, Rettinger G. Humidity and temperature profile in the nasal cavity. Rhinology. 2000;38(4):167–71.
8. Hilgers FJ, Aaronson NK, Ackerstaff AH, Schouwenburg PF, van Zandwikj N. The influence of a heat and moisture exchanger (HME) on the respiratory symptoms after total laryngectomy. Clin Otolaryngol Allied Sci. 1991;16(2):152–6. https://doi.org/10.1111/j.1365-2273.1991.tb01966.x.
9. Rosso M, Prgomet D, Marjanović K, Pušeljić S, Kraljik N. Pathohistological changes of tracheal epithelium in laryngectomized patients. Eur Arch Otorrinolaringol. 2015;272(11):3539–44. https://doi.org/10.1007/s00405-014-3396-5. Epub 2014 Nov 16.
10. Ackerstaff AH, Hilgers FJ, Aaronson NK, Balm AJ, van Zandwijk N. Improvements in respiratory and psychosocial functioning following total laryngectomy by the use of a heat and moisture exchanger. Ann Otol Rhinol Laryngol. 1993;102(11):878–83. https://doi.org/10.1177/000348949310201111.
11. Ackerstaff AH, Hilgers FJ, Aaronson NK, De Boer MF, Meeuwis CA, Knegt PP, Spoelstra HA, Van Zandwijk N, Balm AJ. Heat and moisture exchangers as a treatment option in the post-operative rehabilitation of laryngectomized patients. Clin Otolaryngol Allied Sci. 1995;20(6):504–9. https://doi.org/10.1111/j.1365-2273.1995.tb01589.x.
12. Quail G, Fagan JJ, Raynham O, Krynauw H, John LR, Carrara H. Effect of cloth stoma covers on tracheal climate of laryngectomy patients. Head Neck. 2016;38(Suppl 1):E480–7. https://doi.org/10.1002/hed.24022. Epub 2015 Jul 5.
13. Lorenz KJ, Maier H. Pulmonale Rehabilitation nach totaler Laryngektomie durch die Verwendung von HME (Heat Moisture Exchanger) [Pulmonary rehabilitation after total laryngectomy using a heat and moisture exchanger (HME)]. Laryngorhinootologie. 2009;88(8):513–22. https://doi.org/10.1055/s-0029-1225619. Epub 2009 Jul 30.
14. Keck T, Dürr J, Leiacker R, Rettinger G, Rozsasi A. Tracheal climate in laryngectomees after use of a heat and moisture exchanger. Laryngoscope. 2005;115(3):534–7. https://doi.org/10.1097/01.MLG.0000150417.51835.4F.
15. Icuspit P, Yarlagadda B, Garg S, Johnson T, Deschler D. Heat and moisture exchange devices for patients undergoing total laryngectomy. ORL Head Neck Nurs. 2014;32(1):20–3.
16. Bohnenkamp TA. The effects of a total laryngectomy on speech breathing. Curr Opin Otolaryngol Head Neck Surg. 2008;16(3):200–4. https://doi.org/10.1097/MOO.0b013e3282fe96ac.

17. Bickford JM, Coveney J, Baker J, Hersh D. Self-expression and identity after total laryngectomy: implications for support. Psychooncology. 2018;27(11):2638–44. https://doi.org/10.1002/pon.4818. Epub 2018 Jul 12.
18. Kotake K, Kai I, Iwanaga K, Suzukamo Y, Takahashi A. Effects of occupational status on social adjustment after laryngectomy in patients with laryngeal and hypopharyngeal cancer. Eur Arch Otorrinolaringol. 2019;276(5):1439–46. https://doi.org/10.1007/s00405-019-05378-9. Epub 2019 Mar 29.
19. Bickford JM, Coveney J, Baker J, Hersh D. Validating the changes to self-identity after total laryngectomy. Cancer Nurs. 2019;42(4):314–22. https://doi.org/10.1097/NCC.0000000000000610.
20. Singer S, Meyer A, Fuchs M, Schock J, Pabst F, Vogel HJ, Oeken J, Sandner A, Koscielny S, Hormes K, Breitenstein K, Dietz A. Motivation as a predictor of speech intelligibility after total laryngectomy. Head Neck. 2013;35(6):836–46. https://doi.org/10.1002/hed.23043. Epub 2012 Jun 25.
21. Longobardi Y, Savoia V, Bussu F, Morra L, Mari G, Nesci DA, Parrilla C, D'Alatri L. Integrated rehabilitation after total laryngectomy: a pilot trial study. Support Care Cancer. 2019;27(9):3537–44. https://doi.org/10.1007/s00520-019-4647-1. Epub 2019 Jan 26.
22. Takeshita TK, Zozolotto HC, Ribeiro EA, Ricz H, de Azevedo-Marques PM, Dantas RO, Aguiar-Ricz L. Relation between the dimensions and intraluminal pressure of the pharyngoesophageal segment and tracheoesophageal voice and speech proficiency. Head Neck. 2013;35(4):500–4. https://doi.org/10.1002/hed.22921. Epub 2012 Jan 20.
23. Lorenz KJ. Rehabilitation after total laryngectomy—a tribute to the pioneers of voice restoration in the last two centuries. Front Med (Lausanne). 2017;4:81. https://doi.org/10.3389/fmed.2017.00081.
24. Bozec A, Poissonnet G, Chamorey E, Demard F, Santini J, Peyrade F, Ortholan C, Benezery K, Thariat J, Sudaka A, Anselme K, Adrey B, Giacchero P, Dassonville O. Results of vocal rehabilitation using tracheoesophageal voice prosthesis after total laryngectomy and their predictive factors. Eur Arch Otorrinolaringol. 2010;267(5):751–8. https://doi.org/10.1007/s00405-009-1138-x. Epub 2009 Nov 5.
25. Sokal W, Kordylewska M, Golusiński W. Wpływ wybranych czynników na rehabilitacje logopedyczna chorych po całkowitym usunieciu krtani [An influence of some factors on the logopedic rehabilitation of patients after total laryngectomy]. Otolaryngol Pol. 2011;65(1):20–5. https://doi.org/10.1016/S0030-6657(11)70623-0.
26. Arbutina T, Jovic R, Gasic J, Dragicevic D. Rehabilitation of voice and speech after vocal prosthesis placement. J Otolaryngol ENT Res. 2015;2(4):00031. https://doi.org/10.15406/joentr.2015.02.00031.
27. Galli A, Giordano L, Biafora M, Tulli M, Di Santo D, Bussi M. Voice prosthesis rehabilitation after total laryngectomy: are satisfaction and quality of life maintained over time? Acta Otorhinolaryngol Ital. 2019;39(3):162–8. https://doi.org/10.14639/0392-100X-2227.
28. Bickford J, Coveney J, Baker J, Hersh D. Living with the altered self: a qualitative study of life after total laryngectomy. Int J Speech Lang Pathol. 2013;15(3):324–33. https://doi.org/10.3109/17549507.2013.785591. Epub 2013 Apr 16.
29. Mumovic G, Hocevar-Boltezar I. Olfaction and gustation abilities after a total laryngectomy. Radiol Oncol. 2014;48(3):301–6. https://doi.org/10.2478/raon-2013-0070.
30. Longobardi Y, Parrilla C, Di Cintio G, De Corso E, Marenda ME, Mari G, Paludetti G, D'Alatri L, Passali GC. Olfactory perception rehabilitation after total laryngectomy (OPRAT): proposal of a new protocol based on training of sensory perception skills. Eur Arch Otorrinolaringol. 2020;277(7):2095–105. https://doi.org/10.1007/s00405-020-05918-8. Epub 2020 Mar 21.
31. Ishikawa Y, Suzuki M, Yanagi Y, Konomi U. Effects of nasal airflow-inducing maneuver in total laryngectomy patients based on changes to olfactory test results: a retrospective study. ORL J Otorhinolaryngol Relat Spec. 2022;84(6):429–37. https://doi.org/10.1159/000523794. Epub 2022 Apr 1.

Conclusions

7

The goal of this book is to provide a comprehensive, simple, and practical tool to anyone interested in voice prosthesis. Indeed, it is intended to represent a guide that leads the reader from the beginning—that is when the question arises of how to restore the voice for total laryngectomized patients—to the surgery, up to the in-office management of the voice prosthesis.

The first key message to treasure on is the careful selection of patient: not all patients are the same, not all laryngeal cancers are the same, and not all total laryngectomies are the same.

Then, you should take care that, based on each patient, the surgery for tracheoesophageal puncture can be performed at the same time as the total laryngectomy or later.

The third take home message is the management of complications: when you perform a surgery, whatever it may be, you must be ready to manage intra- and postoperative complications. So, before surgery, you must know any possible complication and, of course, its solution.

The otolaryngologist is also involved in the in-office management and replacement of voice prosthesis.

However, the speech therapist plays a key role in the rehabilitation of the patient undergoing total laryngectomy in terms of respiratory, phonatory, and olfactory recovery.

Indeed, rehabilitating these patients and giving them a voice mean giving them hope and a better quality of life. There is no greater satisfaction than hearing a "thank you" from the patient with own new voice.

C. Saraniti et al., *Voice Prosthesis in Total Laryngectomized Patients*, https://doi.org/10.1007/978-3-031-29654-3_7